The Vegetarian Low-Carb Diet

The fast, no-hunger weight loss diet for vegetarians

The recommendations given in this book are intended solely as education and information. Always consult a medical practitioner before embarking on a diet. The author and publisher cannot accept any responsibility for illness or injury arising out of failure to seek personal medical advice from a qualified doctor.

A note on stevia

Stevia is a natural sweetener that can be used as an alternative to sugar. Stevia is made from a herb and it is extremely concentrated: a speck of pure stevia the size of a sesame seed is equivalent to a teaspoonful of sugar. Stevia has been shown to have a regulating effect on the pancreas. It also helps stabilise blood sugar levels, acts as a general tonic, reduces stomach acid and gas, and inhibits the bacteria that cause dental decay and gum disease.

Stevia in the UK

At the time of writing, it is illegal to sell stevia in the UK. Stevia is available in the US, Canada, Australia and New Zealand. It is possible to purchase stevia on the internet and have it sent to UK addresses.

Copyright © 2005 by Rose Elliot

First published in Great Britain in 2005 by
Piatkus Books Ltd
5 Windmill Street, London W1T 2JA
e-mail: info@piatkus.co.uk

The moral right of the author has been asserted

A catalogue record for this book is available from the British Library

ISBN 0 7499 2584 1

Edited by Kelly Davis
Text design by Paul Saunders

This book has been printed on paper manufactured with respect for the

Acknowledgements

Many people have helped and inspired me in the writing and production of this book, and I'd like to thank them all:

My agent, Barbara Levy, for believing in and supporting the project from the beginning, Judy Piatkus and Gill Bailey, and the whole team at Piatkus, for sharing my enthusiasm and for publishing this book, and Jo Brooks and Kelly Davis for editing the MS so thoughtfully.

There are a number of people whose contributions have been invaluable to me: Cyndi Norman, who runs The Low Carb Forum on the internet; Sara Byk and other contributors to the forum who shared their experiences, tips and recipes so generously and Anna Brian, who gave me such excellent advice on medical and nutritional matters.

Lastly, a big thank you to my family and friends who were so encouraging and supportive, including Chryssa and Carol, and special thanks to my daughter Claire. And finally, a big 'thank you' to my husband, Robert – a traditional vegetarian, no low-carbing for him – for his patience and love and help with the Carb and Protein Counter.

Contents

Introduction

As a cookery writer, constantly thinking and writing about food, not to mention testing, tasting and eating different dishes, it can be quite a struggle to keep slim. So when I heard about low-carb diets, and the large amount of weight people were able to lose on them, while feasting on the foods I love, such as avocado, olives, cheese and raspberries and cream, I was intrigued.

Most low-carb diets, however, seemed to involve eating large amounts of meat and fish, and some even said that they were 'unsuitable for vegetarians'. But I couldn't see why they couldn't be adapted for vegetarians – or even vegans. I began experimenting, on myself and on any other vegetarians who would join in. The more I cooked low-carb vegetarian dishes, the more I liked them. I enjoyed creating recipes with new foods and ingredients, while feeling lighter and more energetic.

At the same time, I read all the books and papers that I could find on low-carbing and I learnt how this way of eating could not only enable someone to lose weight easily and effectively, but could also stabilise blood sugar levels, banish carb cravings, reduce blood pressure and 'bad' cholesterol, and increase energy.

I realised that a balanced, low-carb vegetarian/vegan diet contains many nutritious foods, including soya protein, nuts, seeds, essential oils and generous amounts of vegetables, all of which play an important part in the diet and make it a very healthy way to eat.

So, if you have any of the health problems mentioned above, or if you simply want to lose weight and increase your energy, then this could well be the diet for you. If so, I hope that you'll find it as enjoyable and successful as the many vegetarians of all types – lacto, ovo, demi- and vegan – who have shared their experiences in this book.

The Diet

1

The Vegetarian Low-Carb Diet:
What It Is and Why It Works –
And Why High-Carb, Low-Fat Diets Often Don't …

What It Is

The Vegetarian Low-Carb Diet is a way of eating in which vegetarian or vegan protein foods (such as eggs, cheese, nuts, seeds, tofu, Quorn and soya products) are combined with an abundance of fresh vegetables (including mushrooms, asparagus, spinach, peppers, green beans, cauliflower, courgettes, aubergines, tomatoes, avocados and many more) and healthy fats and oils (such as extra-virgin olive oil and nut oils).

This low-carbohydrate, adequate protein, moderate- to high-fat diet allows the body's metabolic rate to remain high while satisfying appetite and preserving lean body mass. It results in healthy weight loss by lowering insulin levels and this may also have a positive effect on many chronic diseases and health problems.

I believe most people would benefit from this diet, but it could be particularly helpful if you have any of the following:

- High LDL ('bad') cholesterol

- High triglycerides

- Binge eating

- Obesity

- Heart disease

- Impaired glucose tolerance, which may result in, or be classed as:

  - Type 2 ('mature onset') diabetes or

  - Polycystic ovarian syndrome (PCOS)

Many of these symptoms can be associated with hyperinsulinemia (or raised insulin levels in the blood) and may be referred to as 'Metabolic Syndrome', or 'Syndrome X'. This term refers to a cluster of conditions in which the main problem is insulin resistance which results in raised insulin levels in the bloodstream.

The way to heal these conditions is to treat the cause, not the symptom. And the best way to treat the cause – messed-up insulin levels in the body – is a low-carb diet. Cutting out carbohydrates may also improve other conditions, such as anxiety/panic disorder, digestive disorders and irritable bowel syndrome. And losing weight (on this or any other diet) will in itself guarantee a reduction in high blood pressure.

So many vegetarians and vegans experience a tremendous feeling of well-being when they go on the Vegetarian Low-Carb Diet. They find that they have more energy, they feel healthier, and of course they lose weight.

Mary's experience is typical:

'I'm on the Vegetarian Low-Carb Diet because I feel so much better eating like this. I'm not hungry, my joints don't ache like they used to, and I have tons more energy. The best thing of all, of course, is that I'm losing weight! I've already lost nearly 60lb and I've only got another 25lb to go to reach my goal. And, honestly, it really hasn't been that difficult.'

Another successful Vegetarian Low-Carb Dieter agrees:

> 'I found the low-carb diet easy once I got the hang of it. I lost 10lb
> in the first month, followed by a steady weight loss from then on
> – I've lost over 90lb and gone from a size 30 trouser to a size 10.
> Now I don't stand out in a crowd any more and it feels so good.
>
> 'At first, people turned up their noses when I said I was on a "low-
> carb" diet but when they heard that I was vegetarian, they were
> intrigued. They could not understand how it could be done – but
> I am living proof that it can. Now, people I barely know stop me
> to tell me what an inspiration I am to them – and they listen a lot
> more closely to what I have to say.
>
> 'The best thing about the diet, apart from the weight loss, is that
> I'm never hungry and I can eat all the foods I really love: cheese,
> olive oil, nuts, stir-fried tofu and big plates of yummy vegetables.'

Time and again, successful vegetarian and vegan low-carbers say
how much they enjoy the food, how this keeps them motivated, and
how they never feel hungry.

But how can a diet which is low in carbohydrates and rich in
protein and fat – exactly the opposite of the typical, supposedly
'healthy', high-carbohydrate, low-fat diet – be so good for you?
Surely a diet high in protein damages your kidneys and takes
calcium from your bones? And what about cholesterol? Shouldn't
we worry about eating fat?

First of all, just to correct a common misconception, the Vegetarian Low-Carb Diet is not 'high protein': the amount of protein
upon which it is based (60–80g a day) is sufficient to supply normal
needs; it's 'adequate', not 'high' protein. Actually I believe many
vegetarians, who base their diet on carbohydrates, don't get *enough*
protein. There's a limit to how much you can eat, and, if you fill up
with carbohydrates, there isn't much room left for protein. This diet
reverses that. So, although it is true that *high* protein diets have been

associated with a risk of kidney damage in people who have a kidney problem of which they are not aware (as is sometimes the case with diabetics), that is not a problem with this diet because it's *not* high protein.

Furthermore, some studies have shown that eating soya protein actually has a protective effect on the kidneys – another advantage of the Vegetarian Low-Carb Diet. However if you have been told that you have any kind of problems with your kidney function it would be advisable to consult your doctor before undertaking any type of diet. Depending on your personal situation, this diet may still be suitable for you, but you do need to do it under medical supervision.

This diet will not weaken your bones, either. You will lose a bit more calcium than usual at the very beginning of the diet, when you're losing excess water (as you do on any diet). But, after that, your calcium balance will return to normal, with no long-term damage.

As far as eating fat is concerned, yes, we do need to worry about it. But what we need to worry about is getting enough of the right kind of fat. One of the problems with our modern diet is that we are starved of healthy fats – those found in nuts, seeds, eggs and avocados (and fish, for those who eat it) – and this diet puts that right.

Regarding cholesterol, as I've explained later (see pp. 12–13), this is influenced by a number of factors including the amount of insulin in our bloodstream, not just the amount of fat we eat. Having said that, if you're worried about your fat consumption, then this is the low-carb diet for you, because it contains much less saturated fat than a typical meat-based low-carb diet. And the vegan version has none at all, except for the possible inclusion of coconut fat, which, in any case, has some proven health advantages.

Why it works

When we eat carbohydrates – found in sugar, pasta, cereals, bread, cakes, biscuits, fruits, vegetables, lentils and beans – our bodies digest them to form glucose. This circulates in the blood (as 'blood sugar'), providing energy.

This is fine; we do indeed need glucose for energy. However, the amount we get from eating, say, a chocolate bar, a thick slice of white bread or a serving of chips, is normally far in excess of our immediate needs. And if there's a problem with our glucose metabolism, our blood sugar levels can get too high and cause serious health problems such as diabetes.

Fortunately, a normal, healthy body has an in-built mechanism, based on insulin, which regulates the level of glucose in the blood. Insulin is a hormone, or 'chemical messenger', produced by the pancreas. Assuming we don't have diabetes, when we eat sugar, this is what happens:

- The sugar is quickly digested and enters the bloodstream, raising the blood glucose.

- The raised glucose level stimulates the pancreas to release insulin into the bloodstream.

- As the level of insulin rises, it causes the excess glucose to be removed from the blood into the cells, where it is used as energy and any excess stored as glycogen (a stored form of glucose) or converted to fat.

- The blood sugar gradually returns to normal but the level of insulin goes down more slowly.

If we continue to eat lots of concentrated carbohydrates, especially refined ones (like sugar and foods made with white flour), we may become 'insulin-resistant', which means that it takes larger and larger amounts of insulin to reduce our blood sugar. This can lead to diabetes, high blood pressure, raised cholesterol and the increased storage of fat – the group of symptoms known as Metabolic syndrome or Syndrome X.

Excess insulin cannot be treated with drugs, and the usual low-fat, high complex carb diet won't help either: in fact, it will make the condition worse. The more carbohydrates we eat, the more insulin we produce, and the more insulin-resistant we become, which leads to the problems mentioned above.

High levels of insulin in the bloodstream encourage our bodies to turn glucose into fat and store it. However – and here's the good news – low levels of insulin reverse the process: body-fat is released and used as energy. Or, to put it more scientifically, 'in the absence of glucose, which is the body's primary energy source, it will metabolise fat to produce ketones, which in turn can be metabolised to produce energy'.

It's easy to see that, if you're trying to lose weight, getting your body to burn its own stored fat is very helpful. The way to make this happen – to 'switch' your body to fat-burning mode – is to keep your insulin levels as low as possible. And how do you do that? With a low-carb diet!

There are other health benefits too. But, before we look at those, let's just consider the normal 'healthy' high-carbohydrate, low-fat diet and see why it doesn't always work.

Why high-carb, low-fat diets often don't work

The recommendation to eat a diet high in carbohydrate and low in fat came about as a result of studies, carried out from the late 1950s onwards, on the diets of people in countries with a low incidence of heart disease, high blood pressure, diabetes and other common western ailments. This type of diet was supposed to keep us slim and healthy – indeed, 'low fat' has become a kind of health mantra, with a huge manufacturing industry based on it.

But it hasn't worked. Diabetes, high blood pressure and heart disease have reached almost epidemic proportions and – on average – we've just got fatter and fatter. So what's gone wrong?

Let me say right away that I don't doubt that a high-carb, low-fat diet can be healthy, if it's done properly and consistently. However there's a big difference between the way a high-carbohydrate, low-fat diet is followed in the countries studied in the research, and the way we try to put it into practice in modern western society.

In those parts of Asia that haven't adopted westernised food, a high-carbohydrate, low-fat meal might be a large plateful of stir-fried vegetables with boiled rice and a little fish, chicken or tofu, followed by fresh fruit. The 'high-carbohydrate, low-fat diet' that we try to follow in the West is likely to be very different, with far fewer vegetables and much more sugar and refined starch. (Manufactured low-fat foods are often made from refined starches and have sugar added to make up for the lack of fat.)

For many people, it's also a very difficult diet to stick to. As one successful low-carber said: 'Whenever I used to go on a low-fat diet, I absolutely hated it. I just couldn't keep to it, and very soon I'd give up and the weight would go back on again.'

There's no denying that the way we're eating is messing up our insulin and causing many of the other 'Syndrome X' diseases that are on the increase. And, as we've seen, once the damage is done, a very effective way to put it right is to cut out the carbohydrates, as it reduces insulin levels to correct the imbalance.

But aren't carbohydrates essential for health?

Glucose, like protein and fat, certainly is essential to our survival. However, unlike protein and fat, which have to be provided by our food, glucose can be made quite easily by our bodies, using protein and fat. So in fact we can survive perfectly well without carbohydrates. That's what our prehistoric ancestors did, and what some people, such as the Inuits, still do today, remaining free from heart disease and many other illnesses associated with modern civilisation.

Low-carb diets may seem revolutionary, but I can remember my parents dieting like this in the 1960s. They didn't count carbs as such, but they used to talk about 'cutting out starches', and stopped eating bread, potatoes and sugar, of course. No doubt they would have avoided pasta and rice, too, but, strange to think now, they hardly ever used to eat them anyway.

Their meals used to consist of a vegetarian protein savoury – anything from a nut roast, to lentil cutlets or cheese soufflé – and they would usually have two large portions of any vegetables except potatoes or sweetcorn (they liked to have lots of green vegetables). Or for lunch they would have a big salad with yogurt or lemon juice to dress it and grated cheese, devilled eggs or omelette … plus ça change.

Actually, low-carbing goes back even further than that. The first low-carb diet book, *Letter on Corpulence*, was written in 1863, by William Banting, 'as a service to his fellow man', and in fact his name became a verb: 'to bant', meaning 'to diet'. William Banting had himself lost nearly a pound a week for a year by what he described as 'the most easy and comfortable means' and had found his health transformed as a result.

Low-carb health benefits

As you follow the low-carb diet you'll notice other positive effects as well as weight loss: an increase in energy, the disappearance of food cravings and a general feeling of well-being. There will be more benefits, too, of which you may or may not be aware.

The Drs Eades, authors of the excellent book, *Protein Power*, monitor all the patients they put on a low-carb diet. They report that high blood pressure is greatly lowered, or normal, within a couple of weeks, and that there are substantial reductions in blood cholesterol by three weeks. In addition, patients with diabetes and related problems usually have normal, or greatly improved blood sugar levels after just a few weeks.

Reduced cholesterol

You might wonder how a low-carb diet, which doesn't restrict fat, can have such a positive effect on blood cholesterol. This is an important question, because studies show that high LDL cholesterol brings an increased risk of heart disease. (LDL is 'bad' cholesterol, because it's the type which gets deposited in the cells, especially in the artery walls, where it is oxidised and starts to cause plaques which can block the arteries, leading to heart disease. HDL is 'good' cholesterol because it is collected from the cells and taken to the liver for excretion via the bile. So if your HDL cholesterol is high, it means you are getting rid of excess cholesterol.) Another important point about cholesterol is that only 20–30 per cent of it comes from the food we eat. Our bodies make the other 70–80 per cent of it.

Many researchers have shown that cholesterol is increased in most people when they add large quantities of saturated fat to their diet. Note that it increases when they eat the saturated fat in *addition* to their diet. If, however, instead of *adding* the saturated fat to the diet, the researchers *replace* carbohydrates with a corresponding amount of fat, the cholesterol generally does not rise. In fact, it usually falls.

So our cholesterol level is related to the amount of carbohydrates we eat, and, more importantly, the level of insulin required to deal with them. Insulin activates the enzyme that organises the production of cholesterol. Although most of our cholesterol is made by the liver, every cell in our bodies has the capacity to make it.

When insulin increases, our bodies go into fat-storage mode, by converting excess glucose into triglycerides and causing the liver to produce cholesterol. These triglycerides are then transported round the body, where they are deposited into fat cells for storage – and this is also when 'bad' cholesterol gets deposited on the artery walls. So, increased sugar consumption means increased insulin in the bloodstream, which in turn increases the amount of fat stored and the amount of cholesterol in the bloodstream.

When the level of insulin goes down, glycagon (a hormone which works in balance with insulin) is produced. Insulin stores nutrients, whereas glycagon breaks them down. And when glycagon takes over, fat is broken down for energy. The breakdown of the glucose stores, known as glycogen, often releases a lot of water. This is why, on any diet, you get quite a big initial weight loss.

You *can* eat more! The truth about carbs and calories

Is it true that when you go on a low-carb diet you can eat as much as you want and still lose weight?

Well, a calorie is always a calorie *but* protein and fat are harder to break down than carbs. They take more energy – calories – to digest, and some of their calories are 'wasted' in the process.

This effect was shown in a 12-week study conducted by Penelope Greene, PhD, of the Harvard School of Public Health, in 2003. Twenty-one volunteers, all obese and over 50, were randomly assigned either a high-carb, low-fat diet, or a low-carb, high-fat one. In both cases the diets totalled 1500 calories a day for the women and 1800 for the men. A third group had exactly the same food as the low-carb group but the quantities of everything they ate were increased slightly so that they had 300 more calories a day.

The low-fat diet consisted of 55 per cent carbs, 15 per cent protein and 30 per cent fat. The low-carb diet was 5 per cent carbs, 30 per cent protein, and 65 per cent fat.

The food was prepared by an up-market Italian restaurant where the chefs, who had been specially trained, followed the recipes exactly. The food was delicious: there were quiches, some chicken and fish but very little red meat, lots of vegetables and lovely salads, made only with unsaturated oils, and puddings, all carefully prepared, all weighed to the gram and ready for the dieters to collect, every day.

After 12 weeks, participants were weighed and measured, and:

- The low-carb, low-cal group had lost 23lb

- The low-fat group had lost 17lb

- The low-carb group getting 300 calories extra had lost 20lb

Both low-carb groups lost more inches from their weight loss diet – 4 inches at the waist and 3 at the hips – compared with the low-fat group, which lost 3 waist and 2 hip inches.

The experiences of low-carbers bear out these results. Most people on the Vegetarian Low-Carb Diet find that, if they eat whole foods, vegetables, adequate protein and high-quality fats, such as those in nuts, seeds, avocado and olive oil, they lose weight easily without counting calories – and a significant loss of inches is one of the hall-marks of the diet.

How much weight will you lose?

Everyone is different, but one of the joys of the low-carb diet is the encouragingly fast weight loss at the beginning. A number of studies have confirmed the results of Penelope Greene's research described above: people on a low-carb diet lose more weight during the first six months than people on traditional diets. After that, the two groups even up.

It's not uncommon, on the Vegetarian Low-Carb Diet, to lose at least 6–7lb during the first fortnight Carb Cleanse, and some people lose a stone or more, especially if they have quite a lot to lose. After that, weight loss usually steadies to 1–3lb a week.

Apart from the weight loss, one of the big advantages of the low-carb diet is that it's an easy diet to stick to. As Sara, who has lost nearly 100lb doing the diet as a 'demi-vegetarian', says:

'This is the best, easiest diet I've ever been on. I can eat all I want of foods I like, and can eat whenever I'm hungry and worry very little about portions or calories. Once I got used to counting carbs and watching my protein levels, it was all very simple.'

As to how long you can stay on the diet, in my experience, once people try it and discover how good they feel on it, they don't want to go back to their old way of eating. I know people who have stayed on the first phase of the diet, the Carb Cleanse, for many months before moving gently on to the next stage, Continuing Weight Loss, and finally to the Maintenance (or Staying Slim for Ever) phase. And many have continued with this for six years or more. Take Deborah, who says:

'I am 48 and have been vegetarian for some 28 years, and always had tons of energy, although I did find I "slumped" after my main meal. However, five or six years ago, my weight started to creep up, even though I was running 25 miles a week and eating less and less.

'I was diagnosed as having PCOS (polycystic ovarian syndrome), and reading about the condition brought low-carb dieting to my attention. Going low-carb stopped the upward trend of my weight and I have slowly come down about half a stone. But almost as importantly, I don't now feel exhausted after I have eaten. I feel so much better in every way I can't imagine ever eating high-carb vegetarian food again.'

Is there anyone who shouldn't do the diet?

Generally, low-carb diets are not suitable for people with advanced kidney disease because, since the body can only use so much protein, the excess has to be excreted via the kidneys and this can put an extra strain on them. However, as the Vegetarian Low-Carb Diet is adequate protein, rather than high protein, it might be fine.

But you would need to see your GP about it first and obviously only do the diet with his or her approval.

Don't attempt the first two phases of weight loss if you're pregnant or breast-feeding, though Phase 3 (Maintenance), with all the protein, vegetables, nuts, seeds and healthy oils it contains, would be fine.

If you're on medication for high blood pressure, diabetes, or any other related condition, it's essential to speak to your doctor so that he or she can monitor your progress and reduce your prescription as the diet progresses and your condition improves. But don't attempt to alter your dosage yourself. Actually a check-up with your doctor is advisable for anyone starting a new diet, as I've explained on p. 62.

For most people, however, this is a healthy, enjoyable and effective diet. So, now that we've looked at what the Vegetarian Low-Carb Diet is, how it works, and all the health benefits it can bring, let's see how it's done.

CASE HISTORY

Daphne

I'm 40 and I have two children at primary school. I've been obese since childhood – that is, until I discovered the low-carb diet over a year ago and lost over 95lb on it. Throughout my adult life I've never weighed as little as I do now and I can't tell you how wonderful it is. Now I've just got 25lb more to lose to reach my goal weight. At present I'm a (US) Size 10 Gap Bootcut Jean, but I'm aiming for a (US) Size 6!

I've been a vegetarian for over 25 years, starting as a pre-teen, when I would cook for myself. My meals would consist of large portions of grain, or pasta or other starch, a large portion of veggies and a smaller portion of protein. I always liked my cheese and fats.

▶

Once I got the hang of it, I found low-carbing easy. I stayed at 20g carbs a day for most of the time, although now I'm nearing my goal weight I'm being a bit more lenient and including more nuts, a little chocolate (a great low-carb treat) and other things. I eat a good source of protein at every meal but I concentrate more on keeping up my fat intake, which in turn boosts my protein level.

I love eating stir-fried tofu with lots of veggies like eggplant or cauliflower; Greek salad with feta, olives, hard-boiled egg – even some almonds and tofu; lovely omelettes with Swiss cheese or vegetables; spinach or broccoli 'quiche' – egg or tofu based; fried tofu with low-carb peanut sauce; spaghetti squash instead of noodles with a creamy tomato sauce and stir-fried tofu; Indian food like saag paneer, with paneer cheese or tofu – there are so many things. As you can tell, I really love my food and am thrilled that I can really enjoy it on this diet.

I exercise daily and one of my secrets is not to expect too much of myself and burn out. I make myself exercise aerobically a minimum of 30 minutes a day – with it typically being 35 minutes a day. At the beginning of the diet, before I lost my first 60lb, I just walked every day. Now I run, walk, hike, do circuit training, interval training and I mix it up – whatever I feel like doing every day.

If I can do it, anyone can. Don't hold yourself to a timetable or blackmail yourself by saying things like 'if I don't reach 120lb by Thanksgiving, I'll quit' etc; just keep going. I think the important thing is to stay consistent, then you'll succeed.

Chapter 5

How to Do the
Vegetarian Low-Carb Diet

The Vegetarian Low-Carb Diet has three phases: the Carb Cleanse, Continuing Weight Loss, and Maintenance (or Staying Slim for Life, as I like to call it). In this chapter we'll first look at these phases to see what they entail, then find out what you can eat, and how to count carbs and protein. We'll also discover the 12 golden rules for success.

The three phases

Phase 1: the carb cleanse

In the first phase of the diet, carbs are restricted to the lowest level: 20g a day. By restricting carbs to this extent, you can change your metabolism. After the first 48 hours, your body will have used up its supply of stored carbohydrate and will begin burning stored fat for energy instead. You will switch your body from carb-burning to fat-burning and jump-start your weight loss.

As your system is 'cleansed' of carbs, carb-related cravings and mood-swings will disappear – that's why I call it 'the Carb Cleanse'.

If you're like most people you'll experience an increase in energy, a decrease in appetite and – this is the only way I can describe it – an almost euphoric clarity of mind. Oh, and you'll lose a very encouraging amount of weight.

And, no, it won't 'all be water', as critics of low-carb diets claim. Some will be – as on most diets, because that's what happens as part of the metabolic process of fat-shedding – but, after the first pound or two, what you will lose will be fat. As one successful vegetarian low-carber said: 'if it's all water I've lost on the diet, then 50lb and 10 inches off my waist is a heck of a lot of water to lose'!

This phase lasts for a minimum of a fortnight, after which you can move on to the second phase. However, if you're getting on really well with Phase 1, you can continue for longer, making sure that you're getting your 'five portions' of vegetables a day at least (not difficult on the Vegetarian Low-Carb Diet). As I've said before, some people stay on this phase of the diet successfully and happily for many months.

On the other hand, if you find eating just 20g carbs a day too restricting, you could go up to 30g, as I explain on p. 23, and still get good results. I recommend you try starting at 20g carbs and hang on in there if you can. It's only a fortnight, after all – a fortnight that will change your metabolism, your eating habits, your health, and your body, for life.

I like to think of this first phase as a time of cleansing, a time of change, a time of transformation – when the butterfly starts getting ready to come out of the chrysalis!

Phase 2: continuing weight loss

Phase 2 lasts until you reach your goal weight. At the beginning of this phase you gradually increase the number of carbs you're eating, from 20g a day on the Carb Cleanse, to a level which results in a weight loss of 1–2lb a week. For most people, this is around 40–60g carbs a day, which means they can eat delicious meals, with some snacks and treats, while still losing weight steadily.

Phase 3: maintenance

Once you get to the point where you have only 4–5lb left to lose, you repeat the weekly carb-increasing process so that your weight loss gradually stops as you reach your goal weight. Then you will be in Phase 3, using the tools that you've learnt on the diet to stay slim forever, while enjoying wonderful food.

How many carbs can you eat each day, and still stay slim and in control of your eating? This will depend on your own metabolism. For some people it might be 100g or 150g, while for others it may only be 50g or 60g. The chances are that you will certainly be able to include some of the carbohydrate foods you used to love, as I've explained in Chapter 5 ('Continuing Weight Loss'). You will also know exactly how to nip any weight gain in the bud, with a few days on the Carb Cleanse, so that you never again have to 'go on a diet'. What a feeling of freedom that brings.

How to do the diet

To do the Vegetarian Low-Carb Diet successfully, you have to follow three simple principles: cut carbs, add fat and boost protein.

1 Cut carbs

As we've seen, the truth is, whether you're a vegetarian or a meat-eater, when you stop giving your body carbohydrates, you make it start burning fat instead of glucose – and you lose weight. It's as simple as that. You also stabilise blood sugar and insulin, so mood swings and cravings disappear. The metabolic process and the results are the same, whether you're getting your protein from meat and fish or from eggs, cheese, nuts and soya.

So, how do we make the body switch from carb-burning mode to fat-burning, or ketosis, as it's called? It's simple, really: don't give it any carbs! Or just give it the barest minimum. Whereas a 'normal' diet might include 300 or more grams of carbs a day, low-carb diets start you off at anywhere between 20g and 60g a day. Then, when you reach your goal, you increase your carbs again until your weight stabilises.

WHAT IS KETOSIS? AND IS IT SAFE?

Ketosis is the name given to the process that occurs in the body when it has switched to fat-burning mode. Ketones are by-products of the fat-burning process, and the body excretes them through the skin and in the urine.

Ketones are also present when people are starving themselves. In those who are getting plenty of calories from protein and fat but just not eating carbohydrates, ketones simply indicate that they're burning fat for energy. This is absolutely fine. However, in someone with diabetes ketones can be a more serious matter if they are the result of lack of insulin (that is, missed insulin dose in the presence of carbohydrates from the diet). This leads to dangerously high blood sugar levels which can have many physiological consequences.

It's usual to get into ketosis about 48 hours after cutting right back on carbs. Once they have adjusted to this, most people feel wonderful: clear-headed and energetic, with no carb cravings. In fact, ketosis is a natural appetite suppressant and what dieter wouldn't want that? However, it's important to remember to eat regularly and to get enough calories and fat to make the process work safely and effectively.

Once you've experienced ketosis, the feeling is unmistakable. However you can test for it with ketosticks – little strips you can buy at any chemist. Be sure to buy the type that just test for ketones and not the ones for diabetics which test for sugar as well: you don't need this.

You dip a ketostick in your urine and if it changes colour you know you're in ketosis. One word of caution here: if you can't get the ketosticks to change colour, it doesn't necessarily mean you're not in ketosis.

Basically, two types of ketone are excreted, and the ketosticks only pick up one of them. So if you're one of those people (like me) who doesn't excrete much of this particular ketone, the ketosticks won't change colour. But that doesn't mean you're not burning fat and excreting lots of the other ketone.

Some people get an acetone smell on their breath as a result of excreting ketones. Ketosis also acts as a natural diuretic – getting rid of water from the body – when you first go into it. This may be a bit uncomfortable but it doesn't last long and is a sign that your body is healing and transforming itself. And the 'bad breath' that people so often mention with regard to low-carb diets does not seem to be such a problem with the vegetarian version.

The number of carbs you're allowed at the beginning of the diet varies from expert to expert. The Atkins Diet is the strictest, starting off at 20g carbs but another respected and successful low-carb diet, *Protein Power* by the Drs Eades, starts with 30g or even 40g carbs a day (depending on which of their books you read).

Personally, I like to follow Atkins on this and the menus for Phase 1 of the Vegetarian Low-Carb Diet are based on 20g carbs a day. This pretty well guarantees a good weight loss, which is very encouraging. It's actually not that hard to cut your carbs to this level. If you look at the carb comparison chart below, you will see how many carbs you can cut by simply replacing the foods on the left with the foods on the right:

	g		**g**
Slice of toast and marmalade	30	Mushroom omelette	2
Bowl of rice crispies and milk	30	Bowl of Greek yogurt	2
Cheese and chutney sandwich	90	Blue cheese salad	4
Packet of crisps	11	Handful of almonds	3
Apple	17	Bowl of raspberries	6
Glass of orange juice	25	Strawberry smoothie	5
Serving of rice	37	Stir-fried vegetables	4
Baked beans on toast	35	Vegetarian sausages	2
Mars bar	37	Low-carb chocolate bar	3
Vanilla ice-cream	21	Home-made low-carb ice	5
Fizzy drink	20	Sparkling water	0

If, however, you don't get on well starting at 20g carbs, you can go up to a higher level – 30g or 40g carbs – and still be successful. People who have tried both approaches say that in fact they noticed little difference in weight loss whether they started at 20g or 30g carbs a day.

The higher carb level gives more scope for variety and if this helps you to stick to the diet, then that's the right choice for you. The best diet is the one that *you* can stick to.

THE FIBRE FACTOR

Fibre is made up of the natural bran, gums and cellulose that are present in all fruits, vegetables and grains. It's a carbohydrate but it passes straight through our digestive systems and does not raise our insulin levels. Its role in the body is protective: to prevent the sugars in food from being digested too quickly, and to ease the passage of food through the gut.

When the amount of carbohydrate in a food is calculated, fibre is included in the total. However, because it has no effect on insulin

▶

levels, it does not count towards our daily total. We can simply subtract the amount of fibre from the total carbs stated.

So, if the label on the packet says the food contains 12g carbohydrates and 7g fibre, you simply subtract the fibre from the carbohydrates (12 – 7 = 5) to find out how many carbohydrates you need to count (5g in this case). The result is called the 'net carbs', the 'effective carbohydrate content' (ECC) or, the term I prefer, 'usable carbs'. The carb levels given in this book are all usable carbs, unless otherwise stated.

A good food label will tell you both the full carbohydrate content, and the fibre, so that you can do the simple sum described. However, I need to give you a word of warning here. Sometimes the carbohydrates stated have already had the fibre subtracted, so when you take off the fibre you get a 'too good to be true' total. I wish manufacturers would make this clear on the label, but you'll soon get a sense of this.

2 Add fat

When you cut back on carbs, you must add fat, to make up for the lost calories. This is particularly true in the Vegetarian Low-Carb Diet because most of our proteins do not contain fat, unlike meat and fish.

We're all so used to the 'low-fat' mantra that it takes a while to feel comfortable with fat. Yet fat – of the right type – is as essential to health as protein. On this diet, fat is your friend, with one very important proviso: it must be healthy, unrefined and, preferably, organic.

That means no margarine, shortening, hydrogenated or partly hydrogenated fat, harmful 'trans' fats (produced when plant oils are partially hardened), or products containing them. These are not healthy forms of fat.

Butter is fine: although it contains traces of trans fats these particular ones have been found to have beneficial effects. The fat in eggs is fine, as is that in cheese and cream, but try to use organic varieties whenever possible to avoid hormones, antibiotics and pesticide residues which collect in the fat.

While it's perfectly OK to eat some saturated fat on this diet – as long as it's of good quality – it's important to make sure that you're also getting plenty of healthy unsaturated oils. To do this, use olive oil for cooking and buy extra-virgin olive oil, cold-pressed and organic if possible, for dressings.

If you're using any other nut or seed oils, make sure they are also unrefined, cold-pressed and organic, and keep them in the fridge. Use them in salads or as a last-minute addition to cooked vegetables to avoid damaging them by heating. Or get the oils in their freshest, purest form by eating the nuts or seeds themselves, or butters made from them. Although I knew the health benefits of nuts, I was always a bit wary of eating them, because of their fat content, until I discovered the low-carb diet. One of the unexpected bonuses of this diet for me is that I can enjoy eating nuts again!

3 Boost protein

As well as cutting back on carbs, it's important to make sure you're getting enough protein and enough fat. Low-carb diets don't usually stress these points because, for people eating meat and fish, they're not an issue. But vegetarian proteins aren't as concentrated or, for the most part, as fatty, so we do need to think about them.

Protein is vital for growth, for making and repairing tissue and for recovering from infection. Protein is used to make muscle, blood, immune cells and the framework of our bones. It is the main building block of hair, fingernails, ligaments and skin: in fact, protein is essential for life.

So, how much is enough? You can do some complicated calculations based on your lean body mass but for most people it works out at around 60g of protein a day. Aim for a shade more if you're a man, maybe 80g, and if you're very energetic you could go up to 90g.

I must emphasise again, this is not high protein – it's adequate protein. But many vegetarians, who are not eating a low-carb diet, eat quite a bit less protein than this. When they start low-carbing and increase their protein they usually notice a real improvement in their energy levels and general sense of well-being. This was mentioned time and time again by the vegetarian low-carbers I spoke to.

As one said: 'The reason I put on so much weight was because all I really ate before was potatoes, pasta and bread – and I felt tired all the time. When I started the low-carb diet and began eating proper protein foods, I found I had so much more energy. I couldn't believe it. Also, I always felt satisfied. Yes, I did miss my "comfort foods" sometimes, but I just reminded myself how much better I felt. And then there was the weight loss. I lost almost 3 stone and I felt like a different person.'

Where the Vegetarian Low-Carb Diet differs from other low-carb diets is that, while no meat or fish (except oysters) contain carbs, all vegetarian and vegan proteins do, even if in tiny amounts. This means that we have to choose our proteins a bit more carefully, and keep a check on their carb content, to ensure successful weight loss.

So, we're talking about spreading 60–80g of protein throughout the day, for an expenditure of less than 20g carbs, including vegetables, in the first fortnight. Later you can add more carbs so you'll be able to include some of the 'carbier' proteins (such as Quorn) and eat pretty well unlimited quantities of the really low-carb vegetables, as well as the ones that are a bit higher in carbs, and some fruits, too. But for the first fortnight (or longer if you wish – some people stay on this phase, happily and healthily, for months) the aim is to get your protein for as little 'expenditure' of carbs as possible.

To reach a daily total of 60–80g protein, you need to eat 20–27g protein per meal, or 15–20g per meal plus one or two protein snacks totalling 15–20g. This sounds more complicated than it is because, once you're aware of the need for protein, and how much of your favourite foods you need to eat to reach your day's total, it becomes almost automatic. There are so many different foods you can eat, and so many ways to boost your day's protein, as you can see in the following list of vegetarian and vegan protein foods:

	protein	carbs
55g (2oz) Cheddar cheese	14g	0.4g
2 eggs	12g	1.0g
1 scoop micro-filtered whey powder	16g	1.0g
28g (1oz) almonds	6g	2.3g
1 tablespoon peanut butter	4.5g	2.0g
250g (9oz) firm tofu	40g	2.5g
28g (1oz) or 1 scoop soya protein isolate	24g	0g
300ml (½ pint) unsweetened soya milk	11g	1.2g
87g (3oz) 'serving' of Quorn chunks	12g	5.0g
70g (2½oz) 'serving' wheat protein (seitan)	19g	2.5g
2 vegetarian sausages	15g	1.8g
vegeburger 'quarterpounder'	27g	1.8g

When counting up your protein, I suggest that you just add up the main sources, as given above. However there are also small, varying amounts of protein in vegetables, which do add up over the day and help achieve your overall balance, as you'll see in the menu plans (on pp. 73–87). I would aim for 60g protein every day from your main protein foods and count these little extras from vegetables as a kind of safety margin, ensuring that you get enough. See the Carb and Protein Counter (on pp. 312–8) for a full list of foods and their carb and protein contents.

A day's meals

So what does all this look like in terms of a day's meals? It might work out like this.

Breakfast This could be a mushroom omelette, made with 2 eggs and 28g (1oz) grated Cheddar cheese: 21g protein for 3g carbs. Or it could be a bowl of soya or dairy yogurt (see p. 29) with 28g (1oz) grated almonds and a couple of spoonfuls of ground flax seeds (linseeds), again for about 20g protein. Or you could get a really good protein blast to start the day by having a protein shake: soya milk, soya protein isolate powder and peanut butter whizzed to a frothy cream, supplying 40g protein for 5g carbs.

Lunch This could be a big lettuce, rocket or watercress salad (about 1g carbs) with a vinaigrette dressing (no carbs), a handful – about 28g (1oz) – of almonds and 55g (2oz) cheese, if you didn't have that at breakfast. Or you could have your green salad with some thinly sliced tofu, fried in olive oil until crisp and sizzling and served with some mayonnaise for dipping. Either of those would give you well over 20g protein for under 5g carbs. So that brings your protein to 40–60g or more, depending on your choices, for under 10g carbs.

Supper This could be something simple like a vegeburger with cauliflower 'mash', or tandoori tofu with spinach, or steamed broccoli with crisp garlicky seitan, or hot goat's cheese on a leafy salad with walnuts – depending on your choices earlier in the day – each for about another 5g carbs and at least 20g protein. Or, if you've had a lot of protein during the day, you might just like to have a simple, vegetable-based evening meal – perhaps a stir-fry of low-carb vegetables such as bok choy/pak choy and mushrooms, with some garlic and ginger.

What you can eat

Let's look now at the foods you can eat: the proteins, fats and oils, sweetenings, fruits and vegetables, flavourings and drinks in the vegetarian low-carb larder.

Proteins

Eggs

Very low in carbs (about 0.5g per egg) and rich in protein, eggs are a wonderful source of nutrients. Buy organic free-range eggs produced by hens that have been allowed to roam freely and have not been fed antibiotics or other chemicals, which get into the eggs. Feel free to eat as many as you want.

Cheese

Hard cheese is an excellent source of protein and usually pretty low in carbs, but many low-carbers find that their weight loss stalls if they eat too much cheese and other dairy products. On his diet, Dr Atkins limits cheese to 100–115g (3½–4oz) a day and says as a 'rule of thumb' to reckon 1g of carbohydrate for every 28g (1oz) of cheese. This ensures that you don't over-do the cheese, and is a good guide-line though I prefer to count the exact carbs for whichever cheese I'm using (see Carb and Protein Counter, p. 313).

Cream cheese and some low-fat white cheeses are low in carbs; cottage cheese tends to be a bit higher but is perfectly acceptable – certainly from Phase 2 onwards. It's always best to buy organic dairy products if you can because chemical residues, hormones and antibiotics fed to non-organically reared cows get into the milk and tend to collect in the fat.

Many vegan cheeses are too high in carbs and low in protein for this diet. However I know of at least one company making a range of different flavours which are as low in carbs as dairy cheese, though not quite as high in protein. Low-carb vegan cream cheese is quite easy to find. Look around, and read the labels – or make your own easily at home from unsweetened soya yogurt (see below).

Yogurt

Plain, unsweetened yogurt adds useful protein to your diet, especially when combined with other protein foods such as flax seeds (linseeds) and almonds. If you buy real 'live' yogurt (check the label carefully) you really only need to count half the carbs stated. This is because the number given does not allow for the fact that live bacteria will have eaten some of the carbs. Just to be on the safe side, I've gone by what it says on the tub and counted the full number of carbs in the menus and recipe totals. But if you wish you can halve the number of carbs, as indeed I do myself. Whole-milk or Greek yogurt is best for this diet because it's lower in carbs – and so delicious. Look out too, for a wonderful French soya yogurt – or 'soya speciality', as it says on the label – which you can find in good health and organic shops. And you can, of course, make your own yogurt at home quite easily from unsweetened soya milk (or cow's milk, for that matter) using a little bought live yogurt as a starter (see recipe on p. 147).

Nuts and seeds

Whole, roasted, ground, raw, eaten on their own, or mixed with other foods, nuts are both nourishing and delicious. Their protein and carb contents vary, so some are more suitable for low-carbing than others. Almonds are excellent, offering a good quantity of protein for not too many carbs, and Brazils are wonderful value, carb-wise, as well as being a valuable source of selenium, a mineral we all tend to lack. Walnuts, pecans, peanuts, macadamias, pine nuts and hazel nuts are all suitable for low-carbing. Cashew nuts and pistachios are a bit high in carbs but could be included when you get to Phase 3.

Nut butters are wonderful, too. Try to get organic ones without emulsifiers. The oil and solids will separate in the jar, but all you have to do is give it a stir. Really good peanut butter, hazelnut butter and roasted almond butter are so good you could eat them out of the jar. They're also great spread on celery, cucumber or thin slices of raw cauliflower, as a snack, or whizzed up in protein shakes and drinks.

Of the seeds, flax (linseeds), pumpkin, sesame and sunflower are all suitable. Flax seeds are particularly recommended, being high in protein, low in carbs and rich in Omega 3 oil: the best source of this on the planet. Pure seed butters are also excellent –

there are some wonderful organic ones available from good health shops.

Tofu

This is another superb source of protein and so low in carbs that, although you need to be aware of its carb content, you can pretty well eat as much as you want. Again, buy organic tofu, made from non-GMO soya. Carb levels vary slightly from brand to brand, but are so low as to make little difference overall. Watch out, though, for flavoured tofu, which may contain ingredients that increase the carbs. Read the label. Silken and firm tofu are both suitable for the diet. (The recipe section gives more information on how to use them.) I like to use plain, firm tofu for most recipes but some people prefer to use silken tofu for shakes and sauces. Cauldron, which is widely available, is low in carbs.

Tempeh

Like tofu, tempeh (pronounced 'tem-pay') is another traditional fermented protein food from Asia. It's not as low in carbs as tofu, but can be included from Phase 2 of the diet onwards. Read the label and buy one made from soya, rather than from grains, for a lower carb content.

Seitan

Pronounced 'say-tan', this is the protein from wheat, long used in Japan: in fact the name means 'is protein' in Japanese. I love this stuff; it's high in protein and low in carbs, with a chewy texture. You can make it yourself from gluten powder or flour (see recipe on p. 218 – it's really easy!). You can also buy it. Plain, unflavoured seitan can be found in the chill compartment at many good health shops; you may also find organic seitan slices and other delicious products made from seitan. It's often included in manufactured vegetarian protein foods. It's an excellent food, as long as you're not allergic to wheat.

Ready-made vegetarian protein foods

There's an increasing range of ready-made vegetarian protein foods: sausages, fake bacon, burgers, 'mince' and so on. As a dyed-in-the-wool, traditional vegetarian, I never used to go near these. However, since working on this book, I've tried quite a few, and I must say I've been pleasantly surprised, though I wish they weren't quite so salty.

You do need to read labels carefully, because carb content varies greatly. Some are very low-carb and high in protein; others are extremely 'carby' and not a very good source of protein. Also, do buy organic products if you can, because then you know for sure that you'll be avoiding GMOs and trans and hydrogenated fat.

Textured vegetable protein (TVP)

This is our old friend from the 1970s, dried, extruded soya protein, which is still available from health shops in the form of 'mince' or 'chunks'. Again, it's high in protein, and quite low in carbs. Make sure whichever type you buy is GMO-free.

Soya beans (yellow, black and green)

These are an excellent source of protein for not many carbs. The yellow ones are the type used to make soya milk, which in turn is the basis for tofu. Black soya beans can be bought dried from Asian shops. Soaked and cooked, they can be used for recipes such as chilli, black bean soup, bean salad, and so on – anything you'd normally make with beans, in fact. They are suitable from Phase 2 onwards, as are green soya beans, called edamame (pronounced 'ed-a-mammy'), which you can buy frozen in their pods from Asian shops. You cook them for a minute or two in boiling water then drain and serve. To eat, simply suck the beans out of the pods into your mouth. In the US they're available already shelled, frozen: I expect they'll be available here soon, so look out for them.

Quorn

This is a useful protein food, which many vegetarians are happy to use, now that the manufacturers have guaranteed that the egg white used is from free-range eggs. (This does not apply to all Quorn products but it definitely applies to the ones that have the Vegetarian Society symbol.) The carbs in the different products do vary and most of them are rather too high for Phase 1, but they can be a delicious addition to the diet after that. Again I have to say it: read the label.

Protein powders

You can buy micro-filtered whey powder, soya protein isolate powder and rice protein, all unsweetened, and these can be very good for boosting protein. The rice protein is slightly higher in carbs than the others, but useful for variety.

Micro-filtered whey powder is particularly useful for vegetarians because it has the highest biological value of any protein in the world. It also encourages healthy intestinal flora and, according to leading health writer Leslie Kenton, 'helps build a firm, sleek, shapely body better and faster than any other food'.

As these powders are concentrated, it's important to get good-quality ones. Although they may seem expensive, 'per serving' they probably work out at about half the price of buying a cup of coffee – not bad for maybe a quarter of your day's protein. Buy the best-quality micro-filtered whey powder, and GMO-free soya protein isolate: this is the protein that has been extracted from soya. It does not taste as strong as soya flour and is lower in carbs. All these powders are also useful for low-carb baking – I tend to use whey powder and soya protein isolate the most.

Soya milk

This is widely available. Make sure you buy unsweetened – if it says 'plain' it may mean it's unflavoured but could still have sugar added, so check. Be sure to buy organic, which will not be made from GM soya. You don't need to buy 'fresh' soya milk from the chill cabinet: the normal, long-life ones are perfectly fine. Or you can make your own (see recipe on p. 145).

Fats and oils

Butter

Organic butter is best because antibiotics, hormones and other chemicals given to cows become concentrated in the cream of the milk from which butter is made. Ghee (made by melting butter, then heating gently until the solids turn golden, and straining) is a healthy oil for cooking. However, for most cooking I prefer olive oil.

Cream

Cream is allowed but count the carbs: 0.5g for 1 tablespoon double cream, more for single; organic is recommended for the reasons given above. Soya cream is also useful. Although it may contain a trace of sugar, Soya Dream, the kind of soya cream that is quite widely available in the UK, from health shops and some large super-markets, is very low in carbs (it contains fewer carbs than double cream).

Cold-pressed vegetable oils

Extra-virgin olive oil, sesame seed oil and other good-quality veg-etable oils can be used freely. Choose cold-pressed, organic oils for their health-giving properties as well as flavour. I believe olive oil is the healthiest oil to use for cooking, as well as in dressings.

Flax seed oil is an excellent source of Omega 3 oils. Buy it from a health shop where they store it in the fridge, keep it in the fridge when you've bought it, and use it up quickly. Add a teaspoonful to your shakes and salad dressings (never heat it) so that you take about a tablespoonful a day, and you'll never have to worry about supple-menting with Omega 3 oils again.

Alternatively, and I think, even better, you can powder golden flax seeds (linseeds) in an electric coffee grinder (or buy them already ground and store in the fridge). Then you can easily sprinkle them over low-carb cereals or mix them into yogurt or protein 'shakes'. This is how I like to eat flax seed – freshly ground with soya or Greek yogurt, great for breakfast.

Coconut oil, although saturated, has been shown to be a very health-giving oil. It can be used for frying and, in the later stages of the diet, for baking. You can buy virgin coconut oil, which is actually solid until heated, in a tub at good health and organic shops. It's expensive but goes quite a long way and it keeps well. It's also very good to use, incidentally, if you have any kind of yeast infection such as candida because it has been shown to have strong anti-fungal properties.

Mayonnaise

This is unrestricted on the diet if you use the real stuff, which is virtually carb-free. Read the label on the jar or make your own, which takes about two minutes (see recipe on p. 187), and means you can use top-quality, healthy oils.

Sweetenings

Sugar

A teaspoonful of sugar, brown or white, contains about 5g carbs, as does maple syrup; honey and black treacle are about 6g a teaspoonful. In the later stages of the diet, some people find a teaspoonful of strongly flavoured honey, black treacle or real maple syrup useful for flavouring. But these options are clearly not practical when you're trying to keep your day's carbs to 20g or less and break sugar-addiction.

Artificial sweeteners

Most low-carb diet books, including Atkins, warn against the use of aspartame, which can stall weight loss (and, some people believe, is associated with a host of health problems including migraines and vision problems). Instead, they recommend an artificial sweetener called sucralose. This is marketed under the name Splenda and is available in tablet or granular form. The tablets do not contain any carbs but you have to count 0.5g carbs per teaspoonful for the granular type because the 'bulker' in it is carbohydrate.

Splenda is a chlorinated sucrose derivative. There has been no independent, long-term human research on this product. In the view of some leading health experts, the 'hundreds of studies' (some of which show hazards) claimed by the manufacturer were inadequate and do not demonstrate safety in long-term use. Whether you use it or not is, of course, your decision but I don't use it myself and cannot recommend it.

Maltitol and xylitol are other low-carb sweeteners. These are commonly made from corn and, although highly processed, they are all-natural. They pass right through the body without being absorbed, so you don't have to count the carbs. However, they do not agree with some people – they can cause digestive upsets, bloating and flatulence. If you can eat them, they may be useful. But go carefully, starting with small quantities. I think these are fine in small amounts if they agree with you, though I don't recommend them for the first fortnight of the Carb Cleanse. They are included in many manufactured low-carb products (as is sucralose/Splenda). Read the label and decide for yourself what you do and don't want to put into your body.

Stevia

The sweetener I most like to use is stevia. This is about as natural a sweetener as you can get because it's made from a herb. In fact, you can sweeten your tea by just dipping a stevia leaf straight into it. However, it's normally used in the form of a white powder, and that's how I buy it.

Stevia is very, very concentrated: a speck of pure stevia the size of a sesame seed is equivalent to a teaspoonful of sugar. Because it's so concentrated, stevia is often sold mixed with a carbohydrate 'bulker' like rice powder. You can buy it like this, often in little packets, or you can buy it 'pure' as a more concentrated powder, or in liquid form, in a dropper bottle. It's worth trying the different types to see which you like. If you use the type with the 'bulker' added, you will have to add on the extra carbs, though they won't increase the total of the recipe much. Personally, I like the pure stevia powder best. I use it in a shaker so that I can add it in tiny quantities, according to taste.

You can use stevia to sweeten anything, and you can also bake with it, as you'll see in the recipe section. Unlike sugar and artificial sweeteners, it's positively good for you. Stevia has been shown to have a regulating effect on the pancreas. It also helps stabilise blood sugar levels, acts as a general tonic, reduces stomach acid and gas, and inhibits the bacteria that cause dental decay and gum disease.

So, what's the catch? There are two. Firstly, some people don't like the flavour, which is a tiny bit reminiscent of liquorice and ever so slightly bitter, though for me the naturalness of the product outweighs these disadvantages and I've come to really like the flavour. Although pure stevia is about 300 times sweeter than sugar, its sweetness is somehow gentler and subtler than that of sugar and takes a while to get used to.

Secondly, you cannot buy stevia in the UK because it's illegal for anyone to sell it to you. This is because when the European Scientific Commission considered an application for its use it was presented with what health writer Leslie Kenton describes as 'rather bogus data'. Based on this data, the Commission concluded that a test-tube derivative of stevia, known as steviol, 'might produce adverse effects in the male reproductive system and damage DNA'. The EU Standing Committee for Foodstuffs decided that the plants and dried leaves of *Stevia rebaudiana* should not be approved 'due to lack of information supporting the safety of the product'. Since stevia has been grown, studied and used for centuries in many countries, with no ill-effects, and is used by diabetics in many parts of the world and in about 40 per cent of manufactured sweet products in Japan, this was difficult to understand. One can only conclude that the decision had more to do with protecting the sugar and sweetener industries than with concern about people's health and well-being. Unlike sugar and artificial sweeteners, stevia poses no threat whatsoever to human health.

However, stevia can be obtained from the US. There it was classi-fied as GRAS (Generally Recognised As Safe) for decades, and used to sweeten tea, amongst other things. Then the FDA, in a misguided attempt to 'protect' Americans, refused to make it legal. However, after many years of public pressure, it was reclassified as 'Safety Unproven' and it can be found in health shops where it is allowed to be sold as a herb, not as a sweetener. At least you can still buy it there.

Because you need so little, it's light to post, and I find it quite practical to have it sent from the US. I've given details in the Sources and Stockists section of this book (see p. 320).

Stevia is in fact readily available in most countries of the world, including Australia, New Zealand and Canada. According to articles on the Internet, the position is better in these countries and it even looks as if there is a campaign to grow it in Australia, which is fan-tastic news. Readers in these countries will need to make their own enquiries but I think they may be able to buy it at health shops, perhaps classified as a 'food supplement', as in the US.

Fruit and vegetables

All fruit and vegetables contain some carbs. Starchy vegetables, such as potatoes, parsnips, carrots and sweetcorn, contain too many to be included, certainly during Phase 1 and Phase 2 of the diet. But that leaves plenty of others that you can use (see below). Carbs given are for 100g (3½oz), listed in ascending order:

Vegetables
- Endive   0.6
- Chinese leaves   0.6
- Bean sprouts   0.7
- Watercress   0.7
- Chicory   0.9
- Daikon   1.2
- Sweet Romaine lettuce   1.2

- Bok choy/Pak choy   1.2
- Spinach, chopped frozen   1.2
- Spinach leaves   1.4
- Celery   1.4
- Asparagus   1.8
- Bamboo shoots, canned   1.8
- Radishes   1.8
- Mushrooms, white/button   2.0
- Rocket   2.1
- Swiss chard   2.1
- Courgettes   2.3
- Tomatoes   2.7
- Salsify   2.8
- Green peppers   2.9
- Cabbage   3.0
- Cucumber   3.1
- Cauliflower   3.3
- Portobello mushrooms   3.6
- Green beans   3.7
- Okra   3.8
- Broccoli   4.0
- Red pepper   4.0
- Fennel bulb   4.2
- Turnips   4.6
- Spring onions   4.7
- Mangetouts   5.0
- Spaghetti squash   5.1
- Artichokes (globe)   5.8
- Pumpkin   6.0
- Aubergine   6.2
- Onions   8.7
- Butternut squash   9.7
- Water chestnuts (canned)   9.8
- Leeks   12.4

Fruit

- Rhubarb, canned unsweetened   1.0
- Blackberries   4.3
- Frozen mixed fruits (check pack)   5.4
- Raspberries   5.5
- Strawberries   5.7
- Gooseberries   5.9
- Watermelon   7.2
- Cantaloupe melon   7.3
- Loganberries   7.9
- Honeydew melon   8.3

CHOOSE ORGANIC

Organic fruit and vegetables are best because they're grown without artificial pesticides and fertilisers and so contain the lowest possible amounts of potentially hazardous chemicals such as nitrates. No one really knows the effect of these chemicals – or the mixture of them that we get from eating different types of food – but many health experts agree that it's much better to avoid them if possible.

So buy organic when you can – join a local box scheme or shop at a farmer's market, for the best value. But if you can't get organic fruit and vegetables, don't stop eating them! It's still important to use plenty of fresh fruit and vegetables (they're one of the mainstays of this diet). Just do your best, and make sure you wash them very well before use.

Flavourings

- Plain, unsweetened soy sauce (such as Kikkoman, from super-markets as well as Asian stores) is carb-free.

- Wine vinegar and rice vinegar (as long as it's unsweetened) are carb-free but balsamic vinegar is not.

- Plain made mustard (without sugar and extras – read the label) is free.

- A clove of garlic, and a teaspoonful of grated fresh ginger each contain about 1g carbs but you only really need to count these in the early stages of the diet.

- In theory, curry powder and spices may contribute about 1g of carbs per teaspoonful; in practice the amount per serving is likely to be negligible and will only matter during Phase 1 of the diet, if you're being very strict.

- Real vanilla extract and real almond extract are useful in sweet dishes, or to flavour yogurt, giving a pleasant natural sweetness.

Drinks

Non-alcoholic drinks

Caffeine can interfere with the body's insulin balance and can also lead to carb cravings so it's best to avoid drinks containing it, if you can. Decaffeinated tea and coffee are all right; I recommend coffee that has been decaffeinated by the water method, as this leaves no chemical residues. A cup of black coffee, 'real' or instant, with or without caffeine, contains 1g carbs, which you need to add to your day's total.

- Tea, without milk, is free from carbs, as are herb teas as long as they don't contain any sugar – read the label.

- Milk is not allowed, as it's too carby, but you can use unsweetened soya milk (which is low in carbs) instead, or a little double cream diluted with water.

- Sweeten your drinks, if necessary, with stevia or low-carb sweetener.

- Fruit juices and sugary drinks are not allowed because they are too high in carbs. Neither are those sweetened with aspartame, which can stall weight loss (see p. 35).

If you yearn for sweet drinks, try some of the carb-free flavoured waters, or make your own by steeping herbs, such as mint and lemon balm, in a jug of water in the fridge. Or try putting a frozen raspberry, blackberry or strawberry, or a piece of lemon rind or lime rind or some slices of fresh ginger in a glass of fizzy water. This has the added advantage of counting towards your daily 2 litres of water. Hot, cold, fizzy or still, water is the best drink of all, and the more you drink, the better, for this diet.

Alcohol

Alcohol is not allowed during the Carb Cleanse (the first fortnight of the diet). After that, you can have one, or two glasses per day maximum, of *dry* wine with your meals, as long as you count the carbs: 1–1.5g per 30ml (1fl oz), which works out at about 5g a glass.

There is some evidence that drinking a little wine with meals helps decrease insulin levels and this might be one of the reasons why heart disease occurs less in Mediterranean countries than in Britain and the US. Spirits, though technically carb-free, tend to raise insulin, so they are not recommended on a regular basis, and neither is beer, unless you can find a low-carb one.

12 Golden rules for success

1. Count the carbs

Eat no more than 20g a day of carbohydrate during Phase 1. You must count the carbs in your proteins as well as those in the salads and vegetables you eat. Count the carbs in *everything*! You will be able to eat enough – a minimum of 60–80g protein a day and your 'five portions' of vegetables (at least). However, during Phase 1 you will need to choose carefully and keep a note of your carbs.

2. Read labels

Become a skilled label-reader. As vegetarians and vegans, we're used to checking that foods are suitable for us to eat. On this diet, we also have to check the carb content (see pp. 23–4 for how to calculate the 'usable carb count').

3. Beware of 'hidden carbs'

Look out for hidden carbs in things like salad dressings, sauces and gravies. Be careful with prepared salads, such as coleslaw, as they may well contain sugar (or nasty artificial sweeteners), as may bottled teas, flavoured coffees, coffee 'creamers' and many fizzy drinks. Also be very wary of diet products unless they specifically state 'no carbohydrates'. Most of these foods are made for low-fat diets and may be high in carbs. The words 'sugarless', 'sugar-free' or 'no sugar added' are not sufficient. Read the label to find the carb content: that's what you need to know. Also, many products you do not normally think of as foods, such as chewing gum, breath mints and cough syrups, contain sugar, so avoid these too.

4. Eat regular meals

Have three meals a day, including breakfast, and don't skip meals. Eating regularly is an essential part of this diet. Eat until you feel satisfied, but don't over-eat. Most people are amazed at how their desire for food changes when they stop eating carbs. A decreasing appetite is, for many, one of the joys of this way of eating. It doesn't mean you don't enjoy your food just as much – if anything, the opposite – but for most people the desire for food definitely decreases.

5. Don't go more than six waking hours without eating

As your appetite decreases, make sure you don't forget to eat. Never go more than six waking hours without eating, even if it's just a little snack (preferably protein). This will help to ensure the success of your diet by stabilising your blood sugar levels and preventing your body from thinking it's in 'starvation' mode (which makes it hang on to its fat stores, just in case).

6. Get enough protein

Make sure you eat at least 60g protein a day, divided between your meals and snacks. Choose low-carb vegetarian or vegan proteins from the list on p. 27. Low-carb nuts, such as almonds, can be included – count the carbs – and some seeds, particularly flax (linseed), are excellent. It makes sense to spread your protein intake out over the whole day, starting with a protein-rich breakfast and not skipping meals.

7. Make friends with fat

Fat is unrestricted as long as it's 'good' fat, as I've explained on p. 34 – that is, extra-virgin olive oil and other *unrefined* vegetable oils. You can have mayonnaise (as long as it's carb-free), French dressing (extra-virgin olive oil, red wine vinegar, a dash of Dijon mustard if you like, no sugar), butter and double cream, organic if possible.

8. Avoid aspartame

Don't eat foods or drinks that have been sweetened with aspartame, as this can interfere with weight loss. Most low-carb diets allow sucralose (marketed under the name Splenda) or saccharin but be sure to count 1g carbs for every teaspoonful of Splenda – the tablets are carb-free. However I would advise you to be very wary of any artificial sweeteners. My preferred sweetener, carb-free and natural, is stevia, produced from the plant of the same name. (For more about sweeteners, and where to get stevia, see pp. 35–8.)

9. Avoid caffeine

Caffeine can mess up your insulin levels and cause carb cravings (see p. 41), so avoid it if you can. Drink decaffeinated coffee and tea, or herb teas without added sweeteners (read the labels). Avoid coffee substitutes made from cereals that contain carbs. Before I did this diet, I used to keep a pot of coffee on my desk. Now a large jug of hot water has taken its place and I find it a great way to drink most of my daily water. To my surprise, I really don't miss the coffee (and I feel much better). This has been another unexpected bonus of the diet for me.

10. Don't drink alcohol

Alcohol is banned during Phase 1 – wine and beer are too high in carbs and spirits mess with your insulin – but you can drink wine, and a little low-carb beer if you wish, later in the diet (see p. 42).

11. Drink plenty of water

Drink at least 2 litres (3½ pints) of water every day – more if the weather's hot or you're very active. More is fine. Drinking enough water is very important. If you don't drink enough, you may feel tired and the diet won't work as well. Work out a system that enables you to keep a check on how much you've drunk, either by measuring out your day's water and keeping it in a jug in the fridge, or filling up bottles, or whatever suits you. Just make sure you do it – hot, cold, still or sparkling, you need to drink your water.

12. Take your vitamins

Take a good complete multivitamin every day.

Heloise

I'm 52 years old and I've lost 24lb on the diet. I lost 12lb in the first two weeks – I was very strict, carb counting, weighing and measuring. It was a challenge but I felt great and had lost inches as well as pounds. Anticipating leaving my comfort carbs behind was quite daunting when I started, but then I found I enjoyed both the food and the way I felt so much, that I didn't miss them at all. There wasn't anything I disliked about the diet and I didn't go hungry at all.

After two weeks, I continued with the diet but in a more relaxed way, incorporating the odd fish or carb-heavy meal but I do mean odd, as it didn't make me feel good – bloated and stodgy!

I lost a further 12lb in the next six months without really trying, just eating lots of vegetables, and all the fruit I wanted, but hardly ever having potatoes, bread, pasta or rice in any form.

What I liked most about the diet was never feeling hungry – and the yummy recipes, especially the oven-baked frittata which tastes so good and is so convenient for those days when you are on the run. I loved my breakfasts and also enjoyed the Quorn and tofu, and lovely creamy celeriac or cauliflower, whizzed up with olive oil. All my life I've struggled to give up sugar in coffee, and finally I've done it, and still enjoy my coffee. When I started the diet, I put cream in it and it was great – now I have graduated to full-cream milk!

My friends were wonderful and supportive – comments from outside varied from non-committal to scathing … Did it affect me? Not really because I felt so healthy and ALIVE. It's been a gradual process, but it's been such a lifestyle change that it is a permanent way of eating for me now.

My tips to others? Keep a focused attitude of REALLY WANTING TO LOOK AND FEEL GOOD; 'see' yourself as already being the size, shape and beautiful person that you are.

Frequently Asked Questions

I hope I've given you a good idea of what the Vegetarian Low-Carb Diet entails, and all the positive things it can do for you. To clarify it further, here are the answers to some of the most frequently asked questions about the diet.

Surely most people need carbs for energy, especially if they're physically active? Don't athletes do something called 'carb-loading', to give them energy?

Most people do not need carbs for energy, as I've explained in Chapter 1. The body can run very efficiently using the calories in protein and fat, which are slower to digest and give long-lasting levels of energy. Carbs can be useful for someone who really needs a lot of energy, such as a farm labourer or a warehouse stocker. But the problem is that most people take in more calories than they need from 'quick-burn' carbs and don't exercise enough – hence the growing problem with obesity.

Low-carb athletes or serious exercisers can find it helpful to eat a few carbs – say 5–7g, or the equivalent of a teaspoonful of sugar – just before working out. For most people exercising at a normal level, however, that's not necessary, and for endurance sports, a low-carb diet can give better results. A 1974 study of well-trained cyclists showed that those on a diet containing only 7 per cent of carbohydrates were able to pedal nearly twice as long as those whose diet consisted of 74 per cent carbs.

Boosting the energy of an athlete in peak physical condition before a race is of course a specialist subject. The challenge for most people reading this book is exactly the opposite: to burn off an excess of already-stored energy – body fat – and get lean and active, and the Vegetarian Low-Carb Diet can enable them to do this healthily and successfully.

Surely it's not healthy to eat so many eggs? What is the maximum I can eat and stay healthy?

Eggs are a wonderful food and, as long as you're not allergic to them, you can eat as many as you want. Just try to make certain that the ones you buy are organic and free-range. The deeper orange the yolks are, the better.

Some of the foods on the diet seem quite expensive. How can I economise?

Yes, good food costs money, and proteins are more expensive than carbohydrates, but I believe that a healthy diet is an incredibly good investment in the long run. Nevertheless, there are ways in which you can economise. Here are some foods that represent particularly good value for money:

Protein powder (soya protein isolate, whey or rice protein) may seem expensive but actually works out cheap when you realise how much protein you're getting. Having a shake made from these for breakfast, or later in the day, plus some eggs, seitan or tofu, can pretty well supply your day's protein needs, leaving you free to eat whatever seasonal vegetables are available cheaply in the shops.

Eggs, as mentioned, are an excellent, cheap source of protein. Don't economise on quality, though: it's important to get organic eggs in order to avoid unwelcome additives, and free-range eggs for the sake of the hens.

Seitan is an excellent source of protein, provided you're not allergic to wheat. Get some gluten powder, which stores well, and make your own (see p. 218). If you make up a good-sized batch, it will keep well in the freezer, ready for use.

Tofu is not cheap, but so high in protein that a little goes a long way.

Soya milk (unsweetened) is not that cheap so you need to find the cheapest source, perhaps buying in bulk if you've got the space to store it. Or, for rock-bottom economy, if you've got the time, it's also quite easy to make from dried soya beans, which you could buy in bulk (see recipe on p. 145).

Black soya beans can be found, dried, in Asian stores and they work out very cheap. They'd no doubt be even cheaper if you bought them in bulk. They are lovely low-carb, high protein beans, which can be used in many dishes, including chillies, bean salads and burgers.

Yogurt can easily be made at home from either soya milk or cow's milk, saving you a lot of money. Once you get organised, you soon get into the habit of doing it and the results are excellent (see recipe on p. 147). You can also make your own soft cheese by pouring yogurt into a muslin bag and leaving it to drip into a bowl for a few hours in a cool place (see recipe on p. 199).

Nuts and seeds can be bought in bulk if you've got someone who can share the expense and quantity with you and/or you have a freezer in which to store your nuts and seeds. Peanut butter is easy to make but I don't advise you to do so unless you've got a really strong food processor, or you might find your money-saving plans defeated by having to replace your machinery.

Extra-virgin olive oil is not the cheapest of oils, but it's certainly the healthiest. Look out for good deals and offers. It's cheaper in bulk.

Stevia actually works out very cheap. Although you have to get this natural sweetener from the US, which entails forking out for the cost of postage, you only need to use the tiniest amount, so it lasts for ages.

I've got candida. Can I do the diet?

Yes. The fact that the Vegetarian Low-Carb Diet does not contain refined carbohydrates or sugar is a helpful start, as is the use of coconut oil, which has been found to be very effective in clearing candida.

You will have to avoid fermented products, such as vinegar and soy sauce, and of course cheese. Concentrate on tofu, eggs, soya milk (unsweetened, of course) and yogurt (soya or dairy), home-made seitan prepared without soy sauce, pumpkin seeds, sunflower seeds and flax seeds (linseeds), along with plentiful vegetables.

Mushrooms and Quorn are usually banned, at least in the early stages of the diet, as of course is fruit. Nuts are fine, as long as they are freshly cracked, to avoid any chance of mould. Avoid artificial sweeteners, which have been found to feed candida in the same way as sugar does: use stevia instead.

A friend said I shouldn't eat so much soya because it can be dangerous. I'm really puzzled because I thought it was supposed to be very health-giving. Can you explain?

In the last few years there has been much favourable news about soya. Studies have shown not only that it can help fight heart disease and strengthen bones but that it also contains cancer-fighting properties. However some articles have also appeared on the Internet, saying that the positive information about soya is merely hype and that it could even be dangerous. The claims against soya include allegations that it causes nutrient deficiencies, thyroid and reproductive problems, osteoporosis and Alzheimer's disease.

In trying to get to the truth of the matter, there are two important points to bear in mind. Firstly, when a number of studies are done on a particular subject, it's very rare for them all to be in agreement. In most cases there will be the odd 'exception that proves the rule'. It's therefore unwise to jump to conclusions or make recommendations based on just a few studies. By picking and choosing carefully, you can prove just about anything in nutrition. This is why health experts look at all the evidence and pay attention to the totality, rather than to just a few studies.

Secondly, drawing conclusions about human health from studies based on animals can be very misleading. For example, broccoli and other cruciferous vegetables (like cabbage) contain a compound called indole-3 carbinol that can discourage cancer in humans. But in other species, this compound causes cancer. If scientists only looked at the results of the studies in those species, no doubt broccoli and cabbage would be banned.

Many of the claims against soya appear to fall into these two categories: that is, they are based on one or two 'rogue' studies which go against the totality of the evidence; or they are based on animal studies. As John Robbins, who is considered to be one of the world's leading experts on the dietary link between the environment and health, says: 'animal studies are at the very foundation of many of the accusations against soy. But animals are not the same as humans … there is almost no evidence even suggesting they have the same effect in humans.'

John Robbins' clear and informative article, 'What About Soy?', and another equally excellent article, 'Is It Safe to Eat Soy?' by Virginia Messina, MPH, RD and Mark Messina, PhD, are both on the Internet (see Sources and Stockists, p. 322) and give a balanced overview of the claims for and against soya. I suggest you read these articles and make up your own mind, as I have done. Personally, I eat soya all the time with, as far as I can tell, only positive effects. I use soya milk instead of cow's milk, eat tofu in some form or another most days, use both black and green soya beans and also soya protein isolate powder both as a shake and in cooking. But I do make sure that the products I buy are organic or non-GMO, as I feel that is very important.

Can children and teenagers do the diet?

You can certainly adapt the principles of the Vegetarian Low-Carb Diet to suit the needs of children and teenagers. Cutting out sugar, processed food, refined carbohydrates and junk foods are all very positive steps you can take together. And, along with encouraging them to walk as much as possible, this way of eating will help them to lose excess weight gently and effectively.

If you're doing the Vegetarian Low-Carb Diet yourself, either to lose weight or to keep healthy and full of energy, it's easy to adapt meals to suit children. Let them eat unlimited fresh fruit, and give them whole grains (such as brown rice, couscous and organic wholemeal bread) alongside the protein and vegetables that you're eating. If you can get it, try them on low-carb, protein-rich pasta, which can be a better bet for vegetarians than normal pasta because of the protein it contains, with a tomato sauce and grated cheese.

You could also offer them tofu kebabs with peanut sauce and some cooked vegetables or salad; sandwiches made from peanut butter or cheese on wholemeal or home-made Low-Carb Bread (another good source of protein, see p. 294); grilled cheese on Spinach 'Bread' (see p. 159) is also popular, as is Low-Carb Pizza (see p. 255). Vegeburgers or vegetarian sausages always go down well: try them with Turnip Chips (see p. 264) and Easy Tomato Ketchup (see p. 189), instead of French fries, and give them healthy dips like Sesame and Tofu 'Hummus' (see p. 198) with raw carrot, red pepper, cucumber and celery sticks.

Try them on Crunchy Tofu Sticks (see p. 206) or Almond Crackers (see p. 296) with Avocado Dip (see p. 200) – the crisps and crackers add useful protein. Cubes of cheese and hard-boiled eggs make nourishing snacks for vegetarian children; nuts (for children over the age of five), peanut or almond butter spread on pieces of vegetable or apple and pieces of marinated tofu are healthy vegan snacks. If you can, keep plenty of washed crudités – their favourite vegetable pieces, washed, cut and ready to eat – always available for them to snack on.

Eating a filling, protein-rich breakfast is another good habit to instill in children and many of the ideas and recipes in this book are suitable for them. Sara's Hot Cereal (see p. 149), made with soya milk and topped with freshly ground golden flax seeds (linseeds), is a particularly nutritious breakfast for children. Follow this with a piece of protein-rich low-carb toast, perhaps spread with peanut butter, and you're really getting them off to a good start.

Incidentally, sprinkling freshly ground flax seeds (linseeds) over breakfast food is a good way of getting children to eat them, and so get their vital Omega 3 oils. Another way is to stir a teaspoonful of flax seed oil into their peanut butter, but you have to mix this up freshly each time, and keep the flax seed oil in the fridge.

To satisfy a child's sweet tooth, let them have all the fresh fruit they want. Seedless purple or green grapes are particularly sweet, and popular. Slices of apple or pear, segments of orange or tangerine and pieces of melon also go down well. You could try freezing sweet berries (raspberries, blueberries, strawberries) and pieces of melon, then whizzing them with soya milk and a little stevia to make a lovely soft ice-cream. Or give children some Fruity Ice Lollies (see p. 281).

Do try to avoid giving them fruit juice – even the pure type – or at least dilute pure fruit juice with water, as it's a very concentrated source of sugar, albeit from a natural source. If you can get them to enjoy plain water (still, fizzy, hot or cold), you'll be giving them a gift for life.

What is the glycaemic index, and how does it fit in with the low-carb vegetarian diet?

The glycaemic index (GI) is a way of classifying foods according to the speed at which they raise the level of glucose in the bloodstream, with pure glucose registering as 100 on the scale. Ready-to-eat breakfast cereals, mashed potatoes and white rice are also high, while nuts, lentils, spaghetti, barley, most vegetables and oat bran are low. In general, the more processed a food, the higher its GI.

Eating foods with a low GI can be helpful for diabetics and for people wishing to lose or maintain weight. However, the GI of foods varies greatly according to their variety, processing and preparation. For instance, you can increase the GI of cubes of boiled potato by 25 per cent by mashing them. Alternatively, you can lower the GI of potatoes by boiling them in their skins until just tender. Likewise, differences in the ripeness of bananas can almost double their GI.

The aim of both the GI diet and the low-carb diet is to balance the body's insulin output. However, they approach it in different ways. While the low-carb diet is naturally low GI because of the very low quantity of carbs eaten, the GI diet is not necessarily low-carb (although it could be). For instance, a salad made from cooked red kidney beans would be low GI but not low-carb – in fact it would be high-carb!

If you want to follow the Vegetarian Low-Carb Diet I do not recommend that you 'mix and match' with the GI approach while you are in Phases 1 and 2. After that, however, when you reach Phase 3 (Maintenance), you could certainly use the GI value of foods to help you select the most health-giving carbohydrate choices to reinstate. You might find that you can forget all about carb-counting as long as you stick to low or medium GI foods. So you could, for instance, include plenty of low GI fruits such as apples, also lentils and a wide range of pulses.

However, there are two points to watch. Eating more carbohydrate makes it harder, as a vegetarian, to achieve what is normally considered to be an adequate protein level (although you might find that you're fine on less), and eating more carbohydrate, even if it's of the low GI type, can bring back bingeing responses in carb-sensitive people – so watch out for these. For more about the GI, and low or medium GI vegetarian recipes, see my book *Fast, Fresh and Fabulous*.

My local supermarket has started to stock some low-carb foods. Can I use these in the diet?
To be honest, I feel rather wary of these manufactured low-carb foods – I fear 'low-carb' may become the manufacturers' new mantra to replace 'low-fat' and I don't think that bodes well for consumers. One of the great advantages of the low-carb diet has been that few manufactured products were available, so that meals had to be based on fresh, natural foods, prepared at home, with lots of fresh vegetables and healthy oils.

That really is the key to a healthy and successful diet and I think you would be wise to reserve manufactured low-carb foods for occasional use. And do check the labels very carefully. Make sure they really *are* low-carb (you will probably find that many of them are too carby for Phase 1 of the diet), and that you're perfectly happy with the ingredients used – many of the products are likely to contain artificial sweeteners and other far-from-natural ingredients, including cheap, unhealthy fats that you may not want to put into your body.

Another point to bear in mind is that, even though a food may be low-carb, if it's one of your 'trigger' foods (see pp. 114–5) it could start you off on a binge-response just as easily as the normal, carby version … Trigger foods are best banned or binned, whatever their carb content.

This is borne out by the experience of one low-carb vegetarian dieter in the US, where many low-carb products are available. She says:

'I've had to stop using these low-carb speciality products, such as pasta, low carb breads, the baking mixes and all that candy that is supposedly low-carb. At first, I thought I would treat myself a little … then "a little" turned into three months of treats, weight stalls and a small weight gain, and less energy. I found that I developed almost irresistible cravings for the foods, so I had to stop eating them completely and go right back to the Carb Cleanse.

'I have no scientific basis for my opinion; it is just based on my personal experience, but I now think it is a waste of time and money to buy these products. The dollar signs are dancing in the heads of manufacturers and retailers. We who are low-carb eaters are a large base they want to tap. And they know just how to do it. Give us useless, nutrition-less substitutes for pastas, breads, candy, ice-cream, cookies, cakes, etc. The really distressing thing is that these products are now popping up in natural food stores as well.'

I have to say that I agree. Also, remember, whether you're counting carbs or counting calories, it's only possible to eat so much food – and, apart from the odd treat, for maximum health, energy and long-lasting leanness, you want to make your food the healthiest, cleanest and most natural you can.

Is it all right to eat nuts during the Carb Cleanse stage of the diet? Atkins doesn't allow them, but allows other 'free' foods like olives and avocados. Can you explain?

It really is all about carbs. Nuts are fine, even desirable, on the Vegetarian Low-Carb Diet, or pretty well any diet, for that matter (unless you're allergic to them, of course). They are a very nutritious food. But they all contain some carbs, and you must count them. Also, it can be quite difficult to eat just a few and for some people they can be a 'trigger food'. (For more about 'trigger foods', see pp. 114–5.) If this is the case for you, you might be better off using them as an ingredient in, say, a breakfast cereal or main course, rather than as a snack. But if you can keep control of how many you eat, and make sure you count the carbs and add them to your total, you can eat them from the beginning of the diet.

As for so-called 'free foods', Atkins included these in his diet, I believe, to give people an idea of what foods they could eat. He did not mean them to be 'free'. Atkins' diet, like this one, which was inspired by it, depends on counting carbs, and olives and avocado do contain some, even though they may be considered low-carb foods. So, it can't be said too often: count your carbs.

Why isn't fruit allowed on the diet?

Fruit is not included during the Carb Cleanse stage for two reasons. Firstly, even fruits with the lowest number of carbs – raspberries, blackberries, strawberries – are high in carbs compared with vegetables. You get a lot more to eat for your carbs with vegetables than you do with fruit. Secondly, for some people, the taste of sweet fruit can bring on carb cravings.

Having said that, one of the most important principles of this diet is to eat the foods you really love (within the carb allowance, of course). So, if you really, really want some fruit, you could try adding a few raspberries or blackberries, perhaps in a smoothie or whizzed into a creamy breakfast or dessert (see the recipe section). Or you could sweeten rhubarb (fresh, stewed, or a can of unsweetened rhubarb) with stevia or low-carb sweetener and eat that with whipped double cream, or try the Rhubarb Crumble (see p. 284). But do count the carbs!

Once you've completed the first fortnight of the diet, you can certainly include some of the low-carb fruits and, indeed, you are encouraged to do so.

Can I eat low-carb bars? I've heard that they might stall my weight loss.

You can eat whatever you like. Seriously, though, there are a number of points here. First, do make sure that the bars really are low-carb. A lot of manufacturers are climbing on to the 'low- carb' bandwagon and making products that aren't really low-carb. So read the label carefully.

These bars are usually made with sugar alcohols, such as maltitol and xylitol. While these do contain some carbs, they cannot be used by the body but simply pass straight through, like fibre. So the carbs don't count and many of these bars contain only 2–3g 'usable' or 'net' carbs.

The problem is that, for some people, as with other artificial sweeteners, they can stall weight loss. They can also cause stomach upsets, diarrhoea and flatulence. So you need to be a bit cautious. But if you find that you can eat them without any side-effects, and still lose weight, they can be useful for a treat, when you feel like something chocolaty or when you're out and about and can't find anything else to eat that's low-carb. Some of the low-carb bars contain quite a bit of protein so they can even be used as a meal replacement in an emergency.

It's really something you'll have to test out for yourself. Low-carb bars may not be the healthiest things in the world, but if eating an occasional – or even a daily – one helps you to remain on track with the diet and lose weight, then I think that can only be positive. As one successful dieter said:

'I know I probably shouldn't have had low-carb bars but they really helped me keep to the diet, particularly in the Carb Cleanse. I lost over a stone on this so I think you'll agree they didn't interfere with my weight loss. I have a very demanding job and I found that having a low-carb bar at my "low energy" time in the middle of the afternoon really seemed to perk me up. They were also useful for days when I didn't have time to get lunch.'

Hmmm. I'm not sure about using them as a lunch replacement on a regular basis. I'd recommend keeping a tub of protein powder at work and whisking up a shake, or taking a low-carb packed lunch (see p. 161 for several ideas for packed lunches).

If I break the diet and eat a lot of carbs, will I put on loads of extra weight?

This is one of the old wives' tales that you hear about low-carb diets. As I've said before, a calorie is a calorie is a calorie. If you overeat, your body will store the excess calories as fat, whether they come from low-carb or high-carb foods, although as I explained on p. 13 you can get away with eating more low-carb calories.

When you go from eating low-carb to eating high-carb, it may seem as if you've put on extra pounds because carbohydrates absorb more water, but the effect sorts itself out in a day or two.

It's true that people who stop low-carbing do often go back to their old weights, sometimes pretty fast. And if they were gaining weight before, they will continue to gain. But that's because of the food they're eating currently, not because of the low-carb food they ate before.

When they've been low-carbing for a long time, most people can slowly add back carbs, and they will not react badly to them. Some people, however, are always 'carb-sensitive' and get bingeing and hyperglycaemic symptoms (see pp. 4–5) unless they're very careful. That's why, for them, the low-carb diet can be such a life-saver.

Can I use fat-burning products?

I do not know of any so-called 'fat-burning' product which does not have side-effects of one kind or another, some potentially serious. My advice is to be very wary indeed of anything offering you a 'magic' way to lose a lot of weight easily. There is no safe, 'magic' way. The magic lies in finding a diet that works, makes you feel good, and that you can stick to: and I hope and believe the Vegetarian Low-Carb Diet does just that.

CASE HISTORY

Sara

I'm 27 and I've got three young children – my oldest little boy is just 5 years old. I've been doing the low-carb diet for 18 months and I'm very excited because I've lost almost 100lb. I've still got quite a way to go – maybe another 50 or 80lb – but now I've come so far, I know I can do it.

This is the best, easiest diet I've ever been on, but it still hasn't been that easy because my family is not at all supportive and they are constantly telling me all the 'dangers' of low-carb. My husband brings pizza home from work and it's hard to have carby foods in the house and not eat them.

However, it does get easier as you go along. You stop craving those foods so much and you start being able to resist foods you couldn't before. Sometimes they're not even tempting, but other times I'll give in and eat something I really want and you know what? It doesn't taste that good. Maybe the fix is to accept that I'm not perfect. I'm going to mess up sometimes and that's OK. I can try again tomorrow. Heck, I can try again the next time I eat.

I started at 20g a day and then gradually built to between 40 and 50g carbs a day. Most days I aim for about 45g. In the past, going over 40g would send me on a binge, so I had to be very careful, but I don't have to be super-strict about it any more.

I budget out carbs for my sweet treats every day. There's no way I'd be able to stay on the diet if I didn't have my treats. And that's the great thing about low-carb – I CAN have them! They just have to fit into my carb count. In the beginning I used a whole lot of

▶

cream because it was such a rich treat for me then, but now I mostly use soya milk. I'll have low-carb ice-cream made by puréeing frozen fruit with soya milk, sweetened with stevia; herb teas like ginger or mint, sweetened with stevia and a dollop of real cream; hot chocolate made with diluted cream or unsweetened soya milk, cocoa powder and stevia; low-carb cheesecake ...

What I really love about this diet, apart from the weight loss, is that I can have these treats, and also, never being hungry. If I'm hungry, I eat.

Phase 1: The 14-Day Carb Cleanse

We're here – it's time to get started. You know the reasons why the Vegetarian Low-Carb Diet works and why it's healthy; you know the foods you can eat and those you can't; and you know about the three phases of the diet. So now you just need to make a few final preparations.

Preparations

These preparations can really add to your enjoyment of the diet and help you to succeed. Here are my suggestions.

Clear your diary

Although the diet allows for some flexibility in meal-planning, at the beginning you will find it much easier if you avoid dinner parties or lunches where you'll feel under pressure to eat what you're given. Decide when you're going to start the diet and keep the next fortnight as free as you can. Think of this as YOUR time: a time when you're going to nurture and heal your body; a time of transformation, if you like.

It's a good idea to start the diet on a Friday, and plan a quiet weekend. This will enable you to rest if you need to, as your body adjusts. Some people experience 'withdrawal' symptoms, such as headaches or feelings of tiredness and nausea as their bodies adapt to not having carbohydrates and, if they've been drinking a lot of it, caffeine. Treat your body gently and get the rest and relaxation you need, if you possibly can.

Have a medical

Dr Atkins always told people to have a medical check-up before starting his diet and I also recommend that you do this. This will show up any underlying conditions you may have and also tell you your blood pressure, cholesterol and triglyceride levels. You can then have these re-taken when you've been on the diet for a month, and subsequently, so that you can monitor your progress. This diet isn't suitable for people with some conditions (see p. 15).

CASE STUDY

Jane

I'm a vegan and I'm on the low-carb diet to keep my blood sugar stable and for insulin resistance (which might even be borderline diabetes), hormonal problems, CFIDS and fibromyalgia – eating less carbs helps all these – and also because I feel much better eating this way. I'm not as hungry, not as lethargic and just feel generally much better. Also, of course, I'm doing the diet to lose weight! So far I've lost 60lb and I've got about another 20 to go.

I didn't used to eat huge amounts of carbs but I did base my meals around vegetables and didn't worry much about protein … Now I'm eating more protein I'm feeling so much better as well as losing weight steadily.

Weigh yourself

It's also advisable to weigh yourself when you begin the diet, so you've got a starting-point and can record your progress. Opinions vary as to how often you should weigh when you're dieting. It's extraordinary how much what the scales say can affect our motivation. One dieter told me how she went for three weeks without weighing herself, and just knew, from the fit of her jeans, her face and everything about her body, that she had lost weight.

She decided to weigh herself on the morning she was setting off on holiday. She got on the scales, and found that her husband had re-set them to read in kilos, because he had been weighing the suitcases. She had no idea what the kilos meant in pounds and stones but she wrote the figures down and when she was on the plane she worked it out. To her disappointment, she found her weight was exactly the same as it had been the last time she weighed herself. She lost heart and, although she tried to keep to the diet on holiday, her heart wasn't really in it and she felt a nagging disappointment during the whole fortnight.

When she got home and worked out the kilo weight with a calculator she realised that she had got it wrong before and had actually lost 4lb before her holiday. How different she would have felt if she had known this. Yet her weight was just the same, her body was the same; it was just her frame of mind that was different.

So the moral is: know your own mind as well as your body, and use the scales as a positive tool. If you are really happy weighing yourself infrequently and relying on 'the fit of your jeans' – as indeed some of the successful dieters in this book were – then by all means do so.

However what I really advise is that you take the emotion out of weighing yourself by making it a habit to get on the scales every day, preferably first thing in the morning, just like cleaning your teeth. Note down your weight; then, at the end of the week, add up the total amount you've lost, divide by 7 and you'll have your average daily weight loss. If you compare it with the previous week's average weight loss, you'll see immediately whether you're losing, staying steady, or gaining. Taking the weekly average like this also allows for your body's natural fluctuations in weight, according to how much food there is in your gut and, for women, fluid retention at different times in the monthly cycle.

Take your measurements

I'm one of those people who really doesn't like weighing and measuring, so I can understand if you feel reluctant to do this. However, as with the medical tests, taking measurements and writing down the figures at the start of the diet does give you a base-line – and when you've lost all those inches, you'll be glad you did.

Some people like to take photographs, too. If you do this regularly, at monthly intervals, say, or every time you drop 7lb, and stick them in a book, you'll have a visual record which will inspire you and encourage you to keep going.

Set your goals

Goal-setting follows on from the measurements. Once you know where you are now, you can set yourself a goal. It's important that this is both realistic – to keep up your confidence – and exciting, to keep you motivated. However, I recommend that you make your goal something like 'to lose x pounds', or to 'get to my healthy weight', without putting a time constraint on it. The 'must lose x pounds by Christmas' mentality puts unnecessary pressure on you and sets you up for failure, and you don't need that. Make it your goal to follow the diet consistently and to allow your body the time it needs to shed the weight at its own rate – just like the many successful dieters who are featured in this book. What they all have in common is that they trusted the diet and persevered ... that's what it takes.

Start a diary

It's a good idea to keep a diary of your experiences of the diet. Start with your measurements, what you weighed, your goals, your exercise plans, your photos if you've taken them, and update these as you continue with the diet. It can be very useful to note down what you ate each day, what you found helpful, what exercise you actually did, nice things people said to you about your weight loss, rewards you gave yourself, and so on. You could also make a note of your reaction to particular foods, if this was different from usual.

Plan your exercise

There's no doubt about it – this diet works best when you combine it with some regular exercise. This does not have to be a big deal: even a five- or ten-minute brisk walk each day will help to speed up your metabolism and get that fat burning.

A 20- to 30-minute brisk walk, or some other form of exercise you like (swimming is excellent) three times a week, would be good; 30 minutes five times a week would be even better. As you progress with the diet (and the exercise) you'll probably get more active anyway. Weight-training is particularly effective for body-sculpting. Personally, I like to combine some flexibility and toning exercises (yoga or pilates) with walking or swimming – but the secret with exercise (as with diet) is finding what works for you and what you like doing; then there's more chance you'll stick to it.

Tell your loved ones

The people you're close to will need to know about your diet, especially if you live with them and you eat meals together. Their reaction may range from support and encouragement – even joining you on the diet – to criticism verging on sabotage. The most important thing is for you to be clear in your own mind and to stick to your goals. Short of actually sitting you down and forcing food into your mouth, or preventing you from buying the low-carb foods you want, no one can prevent you from doing the diet. It's your body and you have the right to eat as you wish, as long as it's healthy, which the Vegetarian Low-Carb Diet is. I like the saying 'If it's to be, it's up to me': when it comes to it, you are in control.

If your loved ones are worried about you because of scare stories they've read about low-carb diets, get them to read Chapters 1 and 3 of this book, or read them yourself before you tell them of your plans so you're prepared with the answers to their questions.

Clear your cupboards

It's a lot easier to do the low-carb diet – or, indeed, any diet – if you're not constantly being tempted by foods that aren't diet-friendly. If you are on your own, I recommend that you clear your cupboards, fridge and freezer of any sugary, starchy and refined foods. Give them away – or throw them out.

If you're living with other people who want to continue to eat these foods, then obviously you can't take such drastic action. But you can be just as committed – you'll just need a bit more willpower and maybe the co-operation of others in storing (and eating) these foods out of your sight.

Stock up

You can make the diet easier for yourself by stocking up in advance with the foods suggested in the following shopping list and meal plans. If you have time, you could even make one or two of the dishes and freeze them, ready for those times when you're too tired or too busy to do anything other than heat something up. But that's not essential because·I'll be giving plenty of suggestions for quick and easy meals. Just make sure you're stocked up with the basics and ready to go. (For more about preparations to make life easier for you, see p. 131.)

Shopping list

These are all the foods used in the meal plans for the first fortnight. Take a moment to check out the meal plans (see pp. 73–86) and the recipe section before you go shopping, because some of the ingredients may only be used in one or two of the recipes. I've offered lots of choices and alternatives – it's very important to eat the things you like and have time to make – and obviously you only want to buy what you need for these.

Stock up with ingredients you know you'll use. Most vegetables will keep for a few days in the fridge, some longer; eggs, cream, yogurt, cheese and tofu keep well in the fridge, as do olives, fresh ginger and garlic. Nuts, seeds and desiccated coconut are best kept in the fridge if you have room; or you can store them in the freezer and use them almost immediately – they take very little thawing.

If you're going to use gluten powder, you'll have to send away for this (see Sources and Stockists, p. 319), unless it has become available in health shops by the time this book is published. Obtaining stevia, the natural, healthy, carb-free sweetener that I recommend, means a quick trip to New York (hah! only joking) or ordering it, again from the addresses given, allowing a week or so for it to arrive.

While you're shopping, don't forget to buy some good complete multivitamin tablets – not because the diet is inadequate, but as a safeguard, particularly when you're losing a lot of water during the first couple of weeks.

Fresh fruit, vegetables and herbs
Asparagus
Avocado
Basil
Bok choy/Pak choy
Broccoli
Cauliflower
Celery

Chicory

Coriander

Cucumber

Garlic (or use garlic paste, see Store cupboard)

Ginger (or use ginger paste, see Store cupboard)

Green pepper

Lemon

Lettuce (any types you fancy, including Cos/Romaine)

Mushrooms (white closed and large, flat Portobellos)

Olives (black Kalamata and green 'Queen')

Onions

Radishes

Rocket

Salad leaves

Spinach (fresh and frozen)

Tarragon

Tomatoes

Watercress

VEGETABLES – FRESH OR FROZEN?

I prefer fresh vegetables because I find the flavour and texture much better. However, nutritionally, the frozen ones are just as good. And there are some times when frozen equivalents are preferable: frozen chopped spinach, for instance, is best for making some recipes, such as Spinach 'Bread' (see p. 159), where you want the spinach to be pretty dry; and frozen raspberries and other berries are wonderful for using straight from the freezer to make thick, chilled fruity shakes and instant soft-scoop ice-cream. I also like to keep a packet or two of stir-fry vegetables (low- to medium-carb) for those too-tired-to-cook times – yes, cookery writers have them too (see p. 131).

THE PROBLEM WITH PACKAGED SALAD LEAVES

Ready-washed packaged salad can be very convenient when you're in a hurry. As a general rule, I'm not mad about it, though, for a number of reasons. It's not nearly such good value as buying a whole lettuce, and, since it became popular, the variety of whole lettuces available to buy in supermarkets has greatly declined. Also, I don't think it's as fresh or as crisp as lovely, crunchy, whole lettuce. My main problem, however, is that the salad ingredients are washed in strong chemical solutions, some of which, tests have shown, leave residues. Yet, despite this, ready-washed salad has also been found to harbour listeria, salmonella and e-coli bacteria. So, to be safe, you have to wash it again in any case. For all these reasons, I think it's better to buy several whole lettuces, of different types, wash them all (but don't cut the leaves) and store them, interleaved with kitchen paper, in a plastic container in the fridge. They will keep well that way and be ready for instant use when you need them.

Nuts and seeds

Almonds (whole and flaked)

Brazil nuts

Coconut (desiccated)

Flax seeds (linseeds), golden

Peanut butter (without added sugar – usually available from health shops)

Pumpkin seeds

Sesame seeds

Walnuts

Store cupboard

Artichoke hearts (canned)

Basil (dried)

Chilli powder or hot paprika

Cocoa powder

Cumin (ground)

Curry powder

Garlic paste in a jar (to be found with the dried herbs)

Garlic salt

Ginger paste in a jar (to be found with the dried herbs)

Italian seasoning (to be found with the dried herbs)

Mayonnaise (must be virtually carb-free – read the label)

Onion salt

Oregano (dried)

Pepper (black, in a pepper-grinder)

Mustard (Dijon, ready-made)

Mustard (dried)

Raspberry, strawberry and loganberry tea-bags (without added sugar)

Rhubarb (canned, without added sugar)

Salt (preferably low-sodium, potassium-rich)

Stevia (or your choice of low-carb sweetener, see pp. 35–8)

Soy sauce (carb-free)

Tabasco sauce

Tomatoes (canned)

Turmeric powder

Vanilla extract

Vegetarian gelatine powder (usually with the baking things)

Wheat bran (from any health shop and some supermarkets)

Wine vinegar (red is fine for everything)

Dairy

Cream, double

Cheese:

    Blue

    Brie

    Cheddar

    Cream (plain and with garlic and herbs)

    Goat's (Chevre blanc, round, with a soft rind)

    Gruyère

Halloumi

Parmesan (vegetarian)

Eggs (organic, free-range)

Yogurt (whole-milk or Greek, 'live', plain, unsweetened)

Non-dairy

Soya milk (unsweetened)

Soya cream (less than 1.5g carbs per 100ml)

Soya yogurt (plain, 'live', unsweetened, available from health shops or make your own easily from soya milk, see p. 147)

Tofu (plain and smoked)

Other protein foods

Gluten powder (see Sources and Stockists, p. 319)

Soya protein isolate powder (plain, or vanilla, non-GMO, check no carbs)

Vegetarian 'mince', burgers, sausages (frozen or 'chill', as desired, check carbs)

Whey powder, micro-filtered (not more than 1g carbs per scoop)

Rice protein powder (as an alternative to the soya and whey, optional)

Fats and oils

Butter

Flax seed oil (not needed if you include flax seeds in your diet, available from good health shops)

Butter

Olive oil (extra-virgin, organic if possible)

Phase 1: The 14-day carb cleanse meal plans

These meal plans will take you through the first fortnight, the Carb Cleanse. You can make changes to the plans, swapping the days and meals, repeating days and meals that you particularly like, and including your own favourite foods, as long as they fit into your 20g carb allowance. You don't have to follow the days in sequence. And you don't have to eat the full quantity of the foods given (some of the portions are quite generous). Feel free to finish them, or not, as you wish, but don't go hungry.

You don't even have to follow the meal plans at all, if you don't want to; they're really there as a guide, not a prescription. As long as you spread your food evenly throughout the day, eating regular meals and not skipping any, you can plan meals, based on the allowed foods, to your own taste.

An allowance of 20g carbs a day works out at about 5g carbs each for breakfast, lunch and evening meal, with 5g left over for snacks, puddings, soya milk in tea if you want it, hot low-carb chocolate, cream in your coffee. The meal plans are worked out (roughly) on that basis, so the days and the meals within them are pretty inter-changeable. However foods do vary, so look at the carb counts given on the packets, to make sure that they really are very low in carbs.

Just remember to:

- Keep track of your carbs: no more than 20g a day.

- Eat enough protein – at least 60g a day. Boost it with a protein-rich drink if you don't get enough in your meals.

- Get your daily 'five portions' (400g) of vegetables (at least).

- Have three regular meals, and snacks as needed: don't go hungry.

- Include the things you really like – low-carb, of course – this diet is not about deprivation.

- Have fun and enjoy your food.

Day 1

	carbs	protein

Breakfast

	carbs	protein
3 eggs, scrambled with butter, a tablespoonful of cream, salt and pepper;	1.2	19
or Scrambled Tofu (see p. 152);		
1–2 vegetarian sausages;	2	15
½ tomato	1	0.5

Lunch

	carbs	protein
Soft Goat's Cheese and Pecan Salad (see p. 179)	2.4	16.8

Evening meal

	carbs	protein
Asparagus Quiche (see p. 257);	3	25
200g (7oz) spinach, cooked	2.8	7.8

Snack

	carbs	protein
½ avocado with Vinaigrette Dressing (see p. 185)	3.5	4
Total	**15.9**	**88.1**

Well done! You've completed the first day. Treat yourself kindly, and try to get to bed early if you can.

Day 2

	carbs	protein

Breakfast

	carbs	protein
100g (3½oz) Greek or soya 'live' yogurt	2.3*	3.7
with 2 tablespoons ground flax seeds (linseeds)	1.6	4.6
and 15g (½oz) chopped almonds	1.2	3

Lunch

	carbs	protein
Left-over Asparagus Quiche (see p. 257);	3	25
big leafy salad with Vinaigrette Dressing (see p. 185)	2	

Evening meal

	carbs	protein
Tandoori Tofu (see p. 213);	3	40
1 tomato	2.7	0.9

Snack

	carbs	protein
150g (5½oz) no-sugar rhubarb	1.2	1.2
with stevia or carb-free sweetener		
to taste and 1–2 tablespoons unsweetened	0.8	0.3
double cream		
Total	**17.8**	**78.7**

*If you use real 'live' yogurt you only need to count half the carbs stated on the pack (see p. 29).

Some people sail through Day 2, but tiredness and headaches are not uncommon. So treat yourself gently if you feel fragile and try and rest as much as you can. Your body is adjusting – and it will be worth it.

Day 3

	carbs	protein

Breakfast

	carbs	protein
3-egg omelette with mushrooms		
or Flaky Smoked Tofu (see p. 157);	3	20
½ tomato	1	

Lunch

	carbs	protein
Caesar Salad (see p. 174)	4.6	26

Evening meal

	carbs	protein
Spinach and Cream Cheese Gratin (see p. 244);	4	11
½ tomato;	1	0.5
watercress	0.7	

Snack

	carbs	protein
100g (3½oz) plain Greek or	2.3*	3.7
soya 'live' yogurt and 2 tablespoons		
ground golden flax seeds (linseeds)	1.6	4.6
Total	**18.2**	**65.8**

*If you use real 'live' yogurt you only need to count half the carbs stated on the pack (see p. 29).

Another day of adjustment, but you're almost over the worst. By tomorrow I think you'll be feeling a lot better. So hang on to that thought, and rest as much as you can.

Day 4

	carbs	protein

Breakfast

	carbs	protein
High Bran Hot Cereal (see p. 149);	3.1	3.2
whey or soya shake	1	15

Lunch

	carbs	protein
2–3 Devilled Eggs (see p. 193)		
or Tofu 'Egg' Mayonnaise (see p. 183)	2	20
with 100g (3½ oz) green beans	3.7	1.8

Evening meal

	carbs	protein
Griddled Tofu with Mushroom Cream Sauce (see p. 211);	0.5	43
Green salad and Vinaigrette Dressing (see p. 185)	2	

Snack

	carbs	protein
6 large green olives	3	2
Total	**15.3**	**85**

From now on it gets better … That's what most dieters find, anyway. You will begin to feel the benefits of ketosis and those cravings and sugar 'highs' and 'lows' should start disappearing.

Day 5

	carbs	protein

Breakfast

	carbs	protein
Chocolate Energy Shake (see p. 139)	2.6	30

Lunch

	carbs	protein
Low-Carb Vegeburger (see p. 209) **or** 125g (4½oz) smoked or plain tofu, thinly sliced and crisply fried, on a big leafy salad with	3	18
Vinaigrette Dressing (see p. 185) or Mayonnaise (see p. 187)	2	

Evening meal

	carbs	protein
Three-Cheese Cauliflower Gratin (see p. 261);	6.1	25.8
½ tomato;	1	
chicory and watercress	1	

Snack

	carbs	protein
28g (1oz) Brazil nuts	1.4	4
Total	**17.1**	**77.8**

You're doing fine! Keep going. If constipation is a problem, see pp. 90–91, and keep drinking your water!

Day 6

	carbs	protein

Breakfast

	carbs	protein
3 scrambled eggs, or Scrambled Tofu (see p. 152), served on a big (Portobello) mushroom, lightly fried in butter or olive oil	3.4	20

Lunch

	carbs	protein
Cream cheese sandwiches, made with Spinach Bread (see p. 159) **or** Salad Wraps (see p. 161)	5	18

Evening meal

	carbs	protein
2 vegetarian sausages **or** Low-Carb Vegeburger (see p. 209);	3	18
¼ quantity Cauliflower Mash (see p. 260)	5	3

Snack

	carbs	protein
28g (1oz) almonds	2.3	6
Total	**18.7**	**65**

Almost through your first week. Is it getting a tiny bit easier? If your appetite is decreasing, be sure not to go more than six hours without eating something.

Day 7

	carbs	protein
Breakfast		
Peanut Smoothie (see p. 140)	6.3	17.2
Lunch		
Chicory and Watercress Salad with Blue Cheese Dressing (see p. 175)	4.7	25.5
Evening meal		
Quick Curried Tofu (see p. 227);	2	20
½ tomato;	1	
watercress	1	
Snack		
Red Fruit Jelly and 2 tablespoons double or soya cream	1	0.6
Total	**16**	**63.3**

Hurrah! You've completed your first week. You can pat yourself on the back – and maybe give yourself a little (non-food) treat.

Day 8

	carbs	protein

Breakfast

	carbs	protein
100g (3½oz) Greek or soya 'live' yogurt,*	2.3	3.7
with 2 tablespoons ground flax seeds (linseeds)	1.4	9.4
15g (½oz) chopped almonds	1.2	3

Lunch

	carbs	protein
Mimosa Salad (see p. 182) **or** Tofu 'Egg' Mayonnaise (see p. 183), served on lettuce leaves	3.5	14

Evening meal

	carbs	protein
½ packet (115g/4oz) Halloumi, fried or grilled	1.6	24
or bought low-carb vegan burger, served on leafy salad with Vinaigrette Dressing (see page 185);	2	
wedge of lemon	1	

Snack

	carbs	protein
2 celery sticks filled with 1½ tablespoons unsweetened	2	1
peanut butter	3.2	6.8
Total	**18.2**	**61.9**

*If you use real 'live' yogurt you only need to count half the carbs stated on the pack (see p. 29).

Are you managing to exercise? No need to force anything, or push your-self at this stage, but just getting out into the open air and walking for five minutes a day can make all the difference. It's also very soothing.

Day 9

	carbs	protein
Breakfast		
3-egg Gruyère Cheese Omelette (see p. 153)	2	27
or Scrambled Tofu (see p. 152);		
½ tomato	1	
Lunch		
Tomato Cheddar Soup (see p. 163);	6.2	16
radishes, chicory and Mayonnaise (see p. 187)	2	
Evening meal		
Marinated Tofu Stir-Fry (see p. 223)	7.8	27
Snack		
Red Fruit Jelly (see p. 274) with		
2 tablespoons double or soya cream	1	0.6
Total	**20**	**70.6**

Remember this diet isn't about deprivation. Make sure you're including the low-carb foods that you like. But count the carbs …

Day 10

	carbs	protein

Breakfast

Peanut Smoothie (see p. 140)	6.3	17.2

Lunch

Hot Goat's Cheese Salad (see p. 180)	2.2	24

Evening meal

Piece of Oven-Baked Mushroom Frittata, vegetarian or vegan version (see p. 155);	3	15
cooked spinach	2	4

Snack

28g (1oz) almonds	2.3	6
Total	**15.8**	**66.2**

If you're weighing every day, remember it's the week's average that's important, not day-to-day fluctuations. As long as you're doing the diet correctly, the weight will go. Everyone loses at a different rate: one man I know lost nothing for the first 13 days, then dropped 14lb on the fourteenth day!

Day 11

	carbs	protein

Breakfast

	carbs	protein
2 hard-boiled eggs **or**		
slices of Marinated Tofu (see p. 219)	2	20
28g (1oz) Cheddar (or vegan) cheese;	0.4	7.1
28g (1oz) almonds	2.3	6

Lunch

	carbs	protein
Left-over Oven-Baked Mushroom Frittata,	3	15
vegetarian or vegan version (see p. 155);		
watercress	1	

Evening meal

	carbs	protein
Bought vegetarian low-carb		
sausages or burgers **or** Low-Carb	3	15
Vegeburgers (see p. 209);		
¼ quantity Cauliflower Mash (see p. 260)	5	3

Snack

	carbs	protein
28g (1oz) Cheddar cheese	0.4	7.1
Total	**17.1**	**73.2**

Slowly but surely, you're getting there … Don't skip meals; if you're not hungry, have a small protein snack instead.

Day 12

	carbs	protein

Breakfast

Cooked veggie or vegan breakfast:

	carbs	protein
2 low-carb vegetarian sausages;	2	15.5
2 eggs, if desired, **or** Scrambled Tofu (see p. 152);	2	13
½ tomato;	1	
55g (2oz) mushrooms, fried in olive oil	1	1.8

Lunch

	carbs	protein
Sesame and Tofu 'Hummus' (see p. 198)	3	20
with radishes and chicory	2	

Evening meal

	carbs	protein
⅙ quantity Low-Carb Pizza (see p. 255);	4.3	15
green salad with Vinaigrette		
Dressing (see p. 185)	2	

Snack

	carbs	protein
Mug of Low-Carb Hot Chocolate (see p. 141)	2	10.3
Total	**19.3**	**75.6**

Remember to make life as easy for yourself as you can – think ahead, and make sure you've got the low-carb foods you need.

Day 13

	carbs	protein

Breakfast

	carbs	protein
Chocolate Tofu Smoothie (see p. 141)	5	14

Lunch

	carbs	protein
Big leafy salad with		
Vinaigrette Dressing (see p. 185);	2	
tofu (smoked or plain), cut thin and fried crisp;	2.5	40
Mayonnaise (see p. 187) for dipping	2	
A few pumpkin seeds (10g/¼oz)	0.4	1.8

Evening meal

	carbs	protein
125g (4½oz) cooked asparagus spears,		
topped with 85g (3oz) grated Gruyère or	2.5	25.5
vegan cheese		
and browned under the grill;		
leafy salad with Vinaigrette Dressing (see p. 185)	2	

Snack

	carbs	protein
150g (5½oz) no-sugar rhubarb	1.2	1.2
with stevia or carb-free sweetener		
to taste and 1–2 tablespoons unsweetened	0.8	0.3
double cream		
Total	**18.4**	**82.8**

Just one more day to go – I hope you're feeling proud of yourself. Don't forget to keep taking your vitamins.

Day 14

	carbs	protein

Breakfast

	carbs	protein
100g (3½oz) Greek or soya 'live' yogurt,*	2.3	3.7
with 2 tablespoons ground flax seeds (linseeds);	1.4	9.4
15g (½oz) chopped almonds	1.2	3

Lunch

	carbs	protein
Rocket and Parmesan Salad (see p. 178)	3.6	22.3

Evening meal

	carbs	protein
Smoked Tofu Kebabs with Peanut Sauce (see p. 215);	3.3	31
150g (5½oz) broccoli	6	4.2

Snack

	carbs	protein
28g (1oz) walnuts	1.4	2.2
Total	**19.2**	**75.8**

*If you use real 'live' yogurt you only need to count half the carbs stated on the pack (see p. 29).

Congratulations! You've completed the first fortnight of the diet. Your body is now cleansed of carbs and you're on the way to radiant health and permanent slimness. Now go to Chapter 5: Continuing Weight Loss (p. 94) to carry on the good work!

Troubleshooting

Many people sail through the first fortnight and experience only positive effects. However, other people don't feel that great at the beginning and experience some discomforts, especially in the first few days, as their bodies adjust to the new diet. Here are some of the common reactions, and some tips on how to handle them.

Headache, exhaustion, irritability, feeling of 'light-headedness', cold sweats

It's quite common to experience any or all of these symptoms during the first few days of the diet. Your body is missing the quick lift it used to get from sugar and carbohydrates, and also the caffeine (if you used to drink a lot of it).

Rest as much as you can. Drink plenty of water. Don't give up at this stage. These symptoms show that the diet is already working; your body is being cleansed of the effects of carbs, and within a day or two – usually when you wake up on the fourth day after starting the diet, and certainly by the end of the first week – you'll feel like a different person.

If you just can't stand it, boost your carbohydrate level by adding another protein snack – nuts are good, or some hard-boiled eggs or extra vegetables. Then try going back to the 20g level after a day or two.

LOW-CARB SNACKS

- 115g (4oz) plain live soya yogurt has 2.8g carbs
- 150g (5½oz) no-sugar rhubarb has 1.5g carbs (sweeten with stevia or no-carb sweetener)
- 2 hard-boiled eggs have 1g carb

▶

- A whey powder or soya shake has 0–1g carb, depending on brand
- 1 tablespoon peanut butter has 2g carbs
- 28g (1oz) almonds have 2.3g carbs
- 28g (1oz) pumpkin seeds have 1.7g carbs
- 28g (1oz) pecans have 1.2g carbs
- 28g (1oz) Brazil nuts have 1.4g carbs (and are a great source of selenium)
- 28g (1oz) walnuts have 2g carbs
- 28g (1oz) sunflower seeds have 2.3g carbs
- Most cheeses are less than 3g for 100g (3½oz), except for Parmesan (3.2g), Feta (4.1g) and low-fat cream cheese (7g) but try not to eat more than about 125g (4½oz) cheese a day because too much dairy can stall weight loss
- Radishes, chicory and Mayonnaise (see p. 187) or Blue Cheese Dip (see p. 202), see recipes for carbs
- 175g (6oz) avocado has 3.5g carbs

CASE HISTORY

Kelly

I'm self-employed, in my mid-forties, with two sons. I was about a stone overweight but hadn't bothered to do anything about it because I hate dieting and all the self-denial it usually involves. Then my husband went away on a 10-day work trip and I thought I'd take the opportunity – while I was just cooking for myself in the evening – to try the Vegetarian Low-Carb Diet.

I was worried that I'd feel tired and grumpy over the first few days but I actually felt fine. And, once the ketosis kicked in, my energy level definitely went up. Much to my delight, I lost about

▶

half a stone in a week. Now I'm keen to carry on and get down to 9 stone. I love the Spinach 'Bread', and the Cauliflower Mash makes a brilliant substitute for mashed potato. My husband loves curries and we can still enjoy eating them together – I just have Cauliflower 'Rice' instead of Basmati rice.

Over recent years, I've got into the habit of having a couple of glasses of wine most evenings. I thought I'd find it very hard to do without my daily dose of alcohol but, interestingly, I haven't missed it at all. A cup of peppermint tea or Low-Carb Hot Chocolate seems to go down very well instead. All in all, I really don't feel I'm missing out on anything.

Carb cravings

Yes, these may give you trouble, just when you thought you could say 'goodbye' to them forever! Don't worry if you do get carb cravings in the first few days; it's just your body's way of telling you that your reserves of carbohydrates are being used up. Eat whatever protein and fat snacks you want – hard-boiled eggs or crisp, fried tofu dipped in mayonnaise can be very helpful, or even some whipped double cream sweetened with a little stevia or low-carb sweetener.

This phase will only last a day or two. Then you'll experience the wonderful energy-increasing and appetite-suppressant effects of this diet.

Leg cramps

If you get leg cramps, which are quite common in the first few days of the diet, it's probably because you've lost electrolytes (the calcium, magnesium and potassium in your body fluids) as a result of the initial water loss. Be sure to take your daily multivitamins, and keep drinking plenty of water. You could try taking some extra calcium and magnesium – in addition to your daily multivitamin – which can help.

Ascent weakness

Feelings of exhaustion, light-headedness, or weakness and heaviness in the limbs when raising the arms or walking up stairs or slopes (called 'ascent weakness'). This can occur towards the end of the first week or during the second week of the diet. It's not particularly common, although one of the people who tested this diet for me did experience it. As with leg cramps, it occurs because of the loss of electrolytes during water loss.

The answer is water, water, water: make sure you're drinking at least your 2 litres (3½ pints) a day. And don't forget to take a good daily multivitamin with minerals. Take a potassium supplement or use a lo-salt brand of salt in your cooking and at the table – one of those which has most of the sodium replaced with potassium. My favourite one is called Solo.

Make sure you're eating enough: no skipping of meals, remember. You must eat regularly; if you're not particularly hungry, eat a little protein-rich snack like a Devilled Egg (see p. 193), a little cheese or peanut butter and celery, some low-carb Marinated Tofu (see p. 219), or a small handful of nuts. Almonds are particularly good, as they're rich in potassium, and half an avocado, though not a protein food, is another excellent potassium-rich snack.

If there is no improvement, then 20g carbs may be too low a level for your particular metabolism. Move straight on to Phase 2 of the diet (Continuing Weight Loss), and step up your carbs to 25g or 30g a day.

Constipation

Ah, the bane of Atkins dieters! Actually, vegetarian low-carbers don't seem to suffer so much from it because the diet is naturally a bit higher in fibre.

However, it can be a nuisance, especially in the early days as your body adjusts to a new diet. You may have found that this also happens when you go on holiday and eat different foods. Anyway, the answer is simple: eat plenty of fibre.

One of the very best sources of fibre is flax seeds (linseeds), which I've already mentioned (see p. 30). You can take 2–6 tablespoons a day but 2 tablespoons is enough for most people. It's best to grind them up first. That way, the oils are released and you get the full benefit of them, although I have a friend who swears they have no laxative effect unless she eats them whole … If you're the same, have some ground ones too, for the oils.

Wheat bran, which you can buy anywhere, also helps constipation and is very low in carbs. If the flax seed (linseed) on its own doesn't do the trick, try taking 2 tablespoons of wheat bran, too. Or try the high-fibre cereal mixtures in the recipe section of this book.

Another high-fibre food you could try is psyllium husks, which you can buy powdered at a good health shop. You mix it with water and gulp it down (or you can add it to smoothies and drinks but I think it spoils them). Start with 2 teaspoons a day and increase it if you need to. You could also try psyllium husks in tablet form – these seem to work well for some people, and I've also heard that taking one vegan 'multi-detox tablet', containing 'amino acids, vitamin B factors plus fibre and digestive enzymes', available at good health shops, has a magical effect for some people.

One of the simplest remedies I've heard is just to have two large sticks of celery, with a glass of water, every day, preferably at the same time of day. This works like a charm for some people.

And – I've said it before and I'll say it again – make sure you're drinking your water!

Can't count, won't count?

Want to follow the Vegetarian Low-Carb Diet but can't cope with all the carb counting? I recommend carb counting, because you know where you are, you learn so much about different foods, and you can vary your meals by trying new ingredients once you know how many carbs they contain. But, if you find you really can't cope with counting carbs and weighing out portions (even though it does get easier as you go on), you can still do the diet, as long as you're happy to eat simply and quite repetitively. To do the Carb Cleanse this way, just stick to the following foods:

- Eggs, organic if possible: eat as many as you want

- Tofu, plain, organic: so low in carbs that you can eat pretty well unlimited amounts

- Really low-carb ready-made vegetarian protein foods: that is, burgers, sausages, etc, which contain 15–20g protein a serving and only 2g carbs or less

- Salad: pretty well unlimited if you choose Romaine lettuce, endive, chicory, watercress, rocket, celery, daikon, radishes, cabbage

- Vegetables: again, consider them unlimited if you stick to spinach, Swiss chard, bok choy/pak choy, mushrooms, asparagus, celery, daikon, bamboo shoots

- Oils, unrefined, virgin: unlimited

- Some dairy: cheese, cream cheese, yogurt, butter

- Nuts and seeds: you can include them but you must count the carbs in these (see p. 315)

Yes, this approach might be a bit dull, but it's only for a fortnight. Think of this as a time when you can eat simple, healthy foods to cleanse your body, change your eating habits and set yourself on the road to health and slimness.

After the first fortnight you can start adding other foods gradually, as described in the next chapter.

CASE HISTORY

Suzi

I've lost 12lb, and I'd like to lose another half a stone. I've lost weight steadily, though. I wouldn't say it dropped off – maybe because I'm not as young as I was (in my fifties) – but at the rate of 2–3lb for the first couple of weeks or so, and then a steady 1–2lb a week. Even if this isn't that fast, I'm feeling so good about myself and enjoying the food so much that I can be patient.

I found the diet quite easy. I started with 20g carbs a day and have kept to that level pretty much because it seemed to work and I was happy with it. I didn't find it hard to keep up my protein levels because I love tofu – which is a wonderful protein food – and if my protein was a bit low at the end of the day, I'd have a protein-rich drink.

Usually I'll have some kind of egg dish for breakfast, a huge salad with cheese for lunch and a vegetable-based evening meal with maybe a low-carb vegeburger or vegetarian sausages, or tofu, and a big stir-fry. I love to round off my meal with a creamy de-caff coffee.

The best thing about the diet is the feeling of control it has given me. I'm never hungry and I've lost the desire to binge. Also the weight loss, of course.

The most difficult thing is eating out. So many of the 'vegetarian options' are high-carb. I tend to eat some protein, or have a protein shake beforehand, then I can just enjoy the lovely vegetables and salads. It's harder when I go out to friends' houses; they find entertaining a vegetarian challenging enough, let alone a low-carb one! Most people haven't a clue what to do. Still, at least I'll be able to let them have a copy of this book now …

Phase 2: Continuing Weight Loss

I f you're feeling good on the Carb Cleanse, losing weight well, and
have more to lose, there's no reason why you shouldn't continue
eating pretty much as you are for a while longer. Some people stay
at this stage, losing weight steadily and feeling great, for six months
or more.

Just make sure you're getting at least five portions of vegetables
every day, and if you fancy a few berries, you could try including
them, sometimes, too – perhaps in the Creamy Berry Smoothie (see
p. 138), for breakfast or a snack, or the yummy, tofu-based Creamy
Berry 'Yogurt' (see p. 275), which is also great for breakfast, a snack
or dessert: find them in the recipe section. And don't forget your
vitamins!

Increasing your carbs

For most people, gradually increasing the daily carb intake to 30g,
40g, 45g or even higher will give continuing, steady weight loss,
together with the scope for eating a wider range of foods. As one

successful vegetarian low-carber said, 'On 45g carbs a day I can eat more or less unlimited vegetables – all that I want – higher-carb protein dishes *and* a dessert treat such as home-made raspberry ice-cream, and still lose weight steadily.'

You might be able to go higher than 45g carbs a day and continue to lose weight. It very much depends on individual metabolism. The way to find out, as clearly laid out by Dr Atkins, is to increase your carb intake gradually, adding about 5g more carbs a day each week, until you stop losing weight. Here's how it goes:

Week 1: First increase

In week 1, you increase your carbs by 5g a day, so you're eating around 25g carbs. This means you can increase the amount of vegetables you're eating, add a few berries, or simply add one of the '5g carb' foods in the list on p. 97 to your day's meals.

Unless you're really craving something – such as fruit or, dare I say it, a glass of wine – I would recommend you move gently into this phase by eating very much as you have been doing. After all, it's worked for you for the last fortnight. Just increasing the amount and maybe the range of vegetables you're eating (see the vegetable lists on pp. 38–40) is a very good way of moving to a higher carb level.

Your body has just got used to handling around 20g carbs a day. Now you can ease it gently into the next level. If you get any sign of a 'binge' coming on, you may have discovered a food – or a situation – which is a binge 'trigger' for you. Don't eat those foods! See pp. 114–7 for more about trigger foods, binges and how to cope.

At the end of week 1, if you've lost weight, move on to week 2. If you haven't lost weight, then you can stay at this level for another week or two and see what happens, or go back to the Carb Cleanse and continue with that, but including all the low-carb leafy green vegetables you want.

Week 2: Second increase

In week 2, you can add another 5g carbs a day, bringing you up to 30g. You could do this by gently increasing the carbs in each of your day's meals, or you could add an extra two 5g food items, or one 10g one, to your normal meals: a couple of glasses of dry wine, some raspberries and cream or a couple of slices of Low-Carb Bread (p. 294), for instance. Or you could eat a higher-carb evening meal, including ingredients such as Quorn or one of the delicious dishes in the 10g carb list. You can be creative and flexible now, and have fun.

Again, if you've lost weight this week, move on.

Week 3: Third increase

In week 3, you have an extra 15g carbs to 'spend', bringing your daily allowance to 35g. You can continue to add carbs as you have been doing, throughout your day's meals, with more vegetables, selected low-carb fruits, vegetarian protein foods which are higher in carbs, and so on, or you can keep your breakfast, lunch and snacks as they always were, and splurge your extra 15g carbs on a more carby evening meal, such as those suggested in the 15g list below.

Fourth and subsequent increases

If, when you weigh at the end of the third week, you're still losing, you can go up another notch, to 40g carbs a day. Many people find that they continue to lose weight steadily at this level, or even the next, 45g carbs, and this gives enough flexibility to enjoy great meals.

Continue in this way, adding 5g carbs a day each week, until your weight stabilises. To continue to lose weight, simply drop back 5g carbs a day to the previous level, and the following week the needle on the scales will, hopefully, have moved down again.

Your own daily carb level for continuing weight loss

Now you know how many carbs you can eat each day and still lose weight steadily, and all you need to do is to keep to this level until you reach your goal weight.

Your weight loss will continue at a slow, steady pace. Don't try to rush; it's much healthier this way – and remember, we're not talking about a 'quick fix' here. We're talking about permanent weight loss, weight loss which will enable you to reach your goal, and, most importantly, to stay slim forever. No more bingeing, no more energy 'lows', no more yo-yo dieting: just a firm, lean, sleek body, and loads of energy. It's worth being a bit patient to achieve that, don't you think?

Foods you can add

For 5 grams
100g (3½oz) raspberries
2 Nut Muffins (see p. 302)
Rhubarb Crumble (see p. 284) with 2 tablespoons whipped double cream or soya cream
1½ slices Cheese and Almond Bread (see p. 298)
2 slices Low-Carb Bread (see p. 298)
2 slices Instant Microwave Low-Carb Bread (see p. 293)
Bowl of Tomato Cheddar Soup (see p. 163)
Bowl of Creamy Mushroom Soup (see p. 167)
85g (3oz) cottage cheese
Marinated Tofu (see p. 219)
Piece of Mushroom Quiche (see p. 253)
Batch of Chocolate Almond Bark (see p. 306)
200ml (7fl oz) double cream
1 medium plum
Creamy Berry 'Yogurt' (see p. 275)
Piece of Uncooked Strawberry Cheesecake with Strawberry Topping (see p. 283) or Baked Cheesecake (see p. 300)
Piece of Blueberry Pie (see p. 286)

For 10 grams

Raspberry Ice-Cream (see p. 277)

40g (1½oz) cashew nuts

Many ready-made vegetarian protein foods (read the labels)

Serving of Quorn mince, chunks or fillets

Spaghetti Squash with Garlic Cream Cheese (see p. 236)

40g (1½oz) TVP mince (dry weight) as basis for recipes (see p. 32)

Cheesy Portobello Steaks (see p. 210)

Cabbage Tagliatelle with Red Pepper and Artichoke Hearts (see p. 234)

Roasted Cauliflower with Lemon (see p. 267)

Courgette Ribbon Pasta with Mushrooms and Cream (see p. 230)

Large serving of Cauliflower Mash (½ recipe on p. 260)

Batch of Almond Crackers (see p. 296) with cheese

Roasted Red Peppers with Feta (see p. 243)

85g (3oz) blueberries

115g (4oz) melon, any type

1 orange

For 15 grams

Roasted Ratatouille (see p. 266)

Vegetables and Smoky Tofu with Satay Sauce (see p. 220)

Chilli Beans (see p. 228)

Chinese Vegetable Stir-Fry with Garlic (see p. 216)

Cabbage Tagliatelle with Red Pepper and Artichoke Hearts (see p. 234)

Turnip Chips (see p. 264) and Easy Tomato Ketchup (see p. 189)

Parmigiana (see p. 241)

Salad Niçoise (p. 173)

Stuffed Peppers with Soured Cream and Walnut Sauce (see p. 245)

Savoy Cabbage Lasagne (see p. 247)

Tofu Cacciatore (see p. 251)

Large ripe pear

1 medium apple

2 ripe peaches

55g (2oz) plain dark chocolate eg Chocolat Menier: check carbs as brands vary considerably.

Continuing weight loss: tips for success

1 Take it gently

Increase your carb level in weekly increments as described: don't try to rush it. Continue to eat very much as you did in the Carb Cleanse.

2 Count your carbs

Continue to count carbs so that you know where you are and can see how your body responds. Be sure to read the labels on packets and count the 'usable carbs' (see p. 24).

3 Listen to your body

Notice how your body reacts to different foods. A good test is to eat a particular food and then see how your body feels 45–60 minutes afterwards. Do you feel light and energised, or heavy and even 'bloated'? As you eat more healthily, and become attuned to your body, it will give you clear messages about what it does and doesn't like.

4 Stop eating foods that make you gain weight

'Food sensitivity' or intolerance can lead to weight gain, as your body retains more fluid to try and dilute the offending food. Some people are sensitive to wheat and dairy products, for instance. Although the Vegetarian Low-Carb Diet seems to help food intolerance generally, if your weight stalls for no particular reason, be aware of the possibility that you may be sensitive to or intolerant of one of the foods you've been eating. It could be artificial sweeteners, it could be food additives such as MSG. Find out what it is, eliminate it, and the weight will start dropping off again. You can also make this problem less likely by eating food in as natural, unprocessed (preferably organic) a state as possible.

5 Watch out for trigger foods

Watch out for particular foods that start you craving more, or increase your appetite, and also be alert to situations that do the same. For more about this, see 'Coping with Cravings' (p. 115).

6 Keep drinking your water

At least 2 litres (3½ pints) a day, more if you're exercising a lot: don't forget!

7 Keep taking your vitamins

Sorry to sound like your mother, but they really are important.

8 Enjoy your exercise

Yes, I mean it: find a form of exercise you really like – love, even, if that's not asking too much – and just do it. You don't need me to tell you how much better it will make you feel. If you're not already doing it, start today, with just five minutes, and I bet you'll enjoy it. Then increase the time until you're doing a minimum of 30 minutes three times a week. You'll be glad you did and, as you progress on the diet, you'll feel more and more energetic.

Phase 3: Maintenance

Gradually, as you get nearer and nearer your goal weight, your weight loss will most likely slow up. This is inevitable, and it's good, because the longer you're on the diet, the more used you'll get to the kinds of food you can eat, the effect they have on your weight, and the 'low-carb lifestyle'.

In fact, the more slowly you lose the last few pounds and move into Maintenance, the better. Dr Atkins was quite firm about this. He said that this time, when you're within a few pounds of your goal weight but not quite there, is one of the most crucial stages of the whole diet. He even made it the third stage of his diet and called it Pre-Maintenance.

To be honest, I don't think that's strictly necessary. But I do think you need to be aware of the importance of moving very gently and slowly from Phase 2 to Phase 3, and preparing yourself, physically and psychologically, for Maintenance (or 'staying slim forever', as I like to think of it). Statistics show that the majority of people who lose weight gain most of it back again within the first year. You don't want this to happen to you – and it need not. But the preparations you make as you end Phase 2 and enter Phase 3 are crucial.

Your aim is to move seamlessly from 'Continuing Weight Loss' to 'Maintenance'. So, by the time you reach your goal weight, you are already 'in' maintenance – eating the kind of meals you really enjoy and can live with, taking celebrations, restaurant meals, treats and holidays in your stride, and feeling relaxed and comfortable with yourself.

This will enable you to avoid the 'ah, now I can "come off" my diet (and eat myself silly)' mentality: the attitude that you're either 'on' a diet or 'off' a diet, which can lead to bingeing and a creeping-back of all the old eating habits which made you gain weight in the first place. Instead of that, the diet will become a way of life – one that will keep you slim and healthy for ever.

So, here's what you do. Your aim is to slow your weight loss down so that it is, in the words of Dr Atkins, 'almost imperceptible'. At the same time, you want to begin re-introducing some of the foods that you loved before you started the diet, and that you'd like to be able to eat again. What you don't want to do is to upset the balance of your diet, mess up your blood-sugar levels and start putting on weight again. So you need to proceed cautiously, experimentally, trying this and that, seeing what effect it has on your mind and body, and always checking your average weekly weight loss.

If, when you get to within about 7lb of your goal weight, your weight loss is 'almost imperceptible', don't feel disappointed at its slow pace. Instead, realise that your body is doing exactly the right thing and naturally easing you into Maintenance. Continue doing what you're doing, fine-tuning your diet so that it fits your lifestyle and your preferences, and you'll get there.

On the other hand, if at this point in the diet you're still losing steadily, perhaps a pound a week, you now need to slow down your weight loss a little. This may go against the grain – but it will be worth it in the long run. So, you do the same as you did when you were moving from Phase 1 to Phase 2: simply add 5g carbs to your meals for a week, checking your weekly weight loss average, until your weight *almost* stabilises. In doing this, introduce a variety of different foods that you'd like to bring back into your diet, using the Carb and Protein Counter (see p. 312) to guide you.

You can spread your carbs evenly throughout the day, or you can use most of them for a particular carby food that you eat at one meal of the day. At this stage in the diet, you can even 'save' carbs and carry them over from one day to the next, to 'spend' on a special carby treat. You need to be aware that this last approach has its dangers, though. If you find that it is getting you into a 'fasting and feasting' mentality, or that eating your carby treat leads to cravings, then you need to get yourself back on track again quickly (see p. 121).

Everyone needs to work out their own way of moving from 'being on a diet' to 'normal eating' – whatever that may mean. And the ways of doing this are as individual as the dieters themselves. It's a question of finding out what works for you.

You might find, like Heloise (read her inspiring story on p. 46), that you want to continue to eat as you did on the diet but without bothering to count carbs, and with all the fruit that you want, and that you can still keep losing weight very gently and gradually. Or you might find you like to keep to the diet during the week and allow yourself a little more leeway at weekends. Or you could eat low-carb most of the time, with just the occasional carby treat. Or you may find that you can get away with including more carbs in your diet as long as they're natural, high-fibre ones like whole grains, beans and lentils (see p. 54).

I can't tell you which of these approaches is best, because it's a question of what works for you – what you like, what fits in with your lifestyle, and, to get back to where we started, what enables you to go on losing weight, slowly but surely, until you reach your goal.

Whatever you do, the important thing is to be vigilant. As I've said before, this is an experimental time. Keep watching your average weekly weight loss, and if it grinds to a halt completely, or begins to drift upwards again, then you'll know that it's time to cut back. Go back to the Carb Cleanse for a few days if you need to, until you get the weight moving downwards again.

What I will say is that, when you try high-carb foods again, you may be surprised, as are many low-carbers, at how much less you enjoy them than before. It may be hard to believe when you begin the diet but, once you get to this stage, your tastes will almost certainly have changed.

You may find that you have lost your sweet tooth to the extent that even something like a tomato or a piece of red pepper tastes almost like sugar.

You will also have become used to the feeling of lightness and vitality which a low-carb diet gives: the stable energy level; the absence of hunger, cravings, mood-swings, headaches and other symptoms that you had before, and the feeling of being in control.

And you'll have come to love the low-carb food you've been eating on the diet – the gorgeous vegetables, the salads, the avocados, the olives, the cold-pressed oils and dressings, the raspberries and cream, the butter, the cheeses, the nuts and seeds, the spicy tofu. Not to mention the pleasure of eating like this, then stepping on the scales next day and finding you haven't gained an ounce.

Not bad rewards for having the courage and adaptability to try a different way of eating and do a bit of carb and protein counting – don't you agree?

As Julie says:

'I enjoy a variety of foods, and have not counted a single calorie. I was better at counting carbs when I first started but I've been eating low-carb for a while now so I don't really have to track much at all any more. I can go through a day without writing anything down, just eating foods I know are low-carb, and make a pretty good guess at the end of the day where I stand. It's just experience. In the beginning I did write down my carbs and protein but, as I went along, I found I didn't have to do that any more.

'I haven't weighed myself lately, but I seem to be losing: my size 14 jeans are fitting me better and better, anyway, so I must be doing something right. I just want to get back into my size 12s and it doesn't matter what weight I am.'

In a perfect world, by the time you get to your goal weight you'll know how many carbs you can eat each day to feel at your best and not gain weight. In fact you'll probably barely have to count carbs and protein any more because you'll just know what you can and can't eat. You'll have become sensitive to your own reactions, both to foods and situations, and developed your own strategies for coping (having no doubt mastered many of the situations described in Chapter 4).

Yes, you'll no doubt have your ups and downs – literally! But you will know that, if you do lapse, you can always correct the damage – and learn something valuable from the experience so that it will be less likely to happen again in the future.

Vegetarian Low-Carb Diet Survival Guide: Staying Slim For Ever

As any dieter knows, there's a lot more to losing weight and keeping it off than following an eating plan. You also have to go on living your life in the real world – surviving everyday situations, such as cooking for other people, eating in restaurants and dining with friends. Then there are those internal challenges to deal with: food cravings, binges and, every dieter's bugbear, the plateau. Here is a survival guide to help you cope – brilliantly!

Cooking for other people ... and looking after yourself

Cooking for other people, when you're on a diet, is never easy, whatever regime you're following. However, it can be done. One way is to make a main course that everyone can share, along with the vegetables, with extra potatoes, rice or couscous for those who aren't low-carbing.

You can also make a vegetable-based main course that can be cooked, then have different protein foods added to it when it's served. For instance, you could make a beautiful, creamy Coconut Sauce (see p. 192) and then serve it over, say, Marinated Tofu (see p. 219), or Quorn nuggets, or chicken-flavoured soya protein – even chicken itself, for those who eat it. These proteins can be cooked separately while the sauce is cooking. Ratatouille works well as a meal basis like this, too, as do Roasted Vegetables (see p. 265).

When you're cooking for a number of different tastes, the freezer makes life a lot easier. Foods can be frozen in portions ready for almost instant use, especially if you have a microwave. A good Nut Roast (see p. 249) – which I and all my family and friends love – can be very useful here because it can be frozen in slices, is great hot or cold, and packed with protein. If you've got people in your house with nut allergies, then clearly that won't do. But there are ever-increasing numbers of low-carb vegetarian protein foods to choose from. Just check the carbs and make sure they're free of GMOs and trans fats. You're safe on these counts if you choose organic.

Thinking ahead like this, about the occasion, and the foods that you are going to eat and provide for others, can make a big difference to your stress level and even to your success with the diet. It's really worth taking the time to make some simple meal plans for the week and then to see that you have the ingredients in stock – *including* the low-carb ones that *you* need. And if you've prepared some food in advance, as mentioned above, and described on pp. 131–3, making a meal, perhaps when you're tired and hungry, is so much easier.

For instance, having some of your own Low-Carb Pizza (see p. 255) in the freezer, ready to pop into the oven when you put in the normal pizza for the rest of the party, can make all the difference between staying on the diet successfully and having 'just one (fatal) bite' of theirs. So can having the ingredients available to whisk yourself up some delicious Raspberry Ice-Cream (see p. 277) when they start serving out the Häagen-Dazs, or some Low-Carb Bread (see p. 294), Almond Crackers (see p. 296) or other low-carb replacement for the foods the rest are eating.

This may seem like a lot of effort – and if you're always thinking about other people, maybe you're not used to taking trouble over your own food or even thinking about your own needs. But it's all about caring for yourself. Aren't these the very things you'd do for a loved one, if they were following the diet? So why not do them for yourself? At risk of sounding like a self-help manual, I do believe that to do a diet successfully, and to keep the weight off permanently, you need to consider yourself, your feelings and your needs, and allow for these in your plans. This really is important.

Eating out

Eating out as a low-carb vegetarian is a bit like eating out as a vegetarian used to be, some years ago, before restaurants started to include 'vegetarian options' in their menus. Now, although the range of dishes offered tends to be rather small, it's quite easy for vegetarians to eat out.

But it's not so easy for low-carb vegetarians because the 'vegetarian options' are usually based on pasta, rice, potatoes or other starchy foods. Sometimes it's even hard to get that simplest of foods, an omelette, which, ironically, was what vegetarians were offered all the time when I was growing up.

Getting what you want in a restaurant really follows on from what I've already said – it starts with valuing yourself and recognising that your needs are important. That's not easy if, like the majority of people with a weight problem, you are used to putting other people first, saying that what you need 'isn't important', and just 'fitting in'. Well, your needs *are* important, and the more you recognise and voice them, the more chance you have of being successful with the diet and remaining slim.

You don't have to be a pain to get what you want. You just need, firstly, to be aware of what it *is* you want, and secondly to have the confidence and courage to ask for it. Yes, just ask: no apologies, no grovelling, no drama: just a simple request. And, if you make this request with the assumption that it's reasonable and will be granted (which in my experience it pretty well always is), no one will think the worse of you.

Of course, as with cooking for others, it really helps if you can plan ahead. Choose a restaurant which is likely to be able to give you what you want – and where you won't be horrendously tempted by your favourite carby foods – and go at a time when the restaurant staff aren't rushed off their feet. Think about the problems or challenges you might encounter and what you're going to do to overcome them. Make up your mind that you're going to stick to your diet – just like the successful dieters in this book did – and then do it.

You'll be so pleased with yourself afterwards – and justifiably so. But the best bit – apart from what the scales will tell you, and also knowing that you can live in the real world and survive as a low-carb dieter – is that every time you do this, the easier (and more fun – yes, really) it will be. And you will be getting stronger and more powerful, and more likely to succeed with the diet – and with life. Don't let anyone destroy your dreams or dash your spirit!

But back to the restaurant: you'll need to study the menu carefully, ask questions about ingredients (e.g. Does the dressing include sugar?) and then probably pick out the bits you can eat and leave the rest (depending on how successful you've been at getting something low-carb). Ask for extra vegetables or salad instead of potatoes and pass on the bread, of course.

With any luck, there will be strawberries or other berries for pudding (make sure there's no added sugar) or fruit salad (OK if made without sugar) or even melon from the starters at a pinch – all with a generous amount of cream if you wish. Otherwise, if there's no suitable pudding, coffee with cream, or a cappuccino, or a nice strong mint tea, can often fill the gap. And if you eat cheese, 'biscuits and cheese', without the biscuits, is an easy option.

AT RESTAURANTS – THINGS TO WATCH OUT FOR

- Bread – wave the bread basket away before you're tempted
- Flour-thickened sauces
- Flour-thickened soups
- Sugar in dressings, sauces and on fruit
- Croûtons in salads
- Breadcrumb coatings and toppings

A really good Indian restaurant is probably one of the best places to get a low-carb vegetarian meal. Although you need to watch out for channa (chick peas) and lentil dal, which are a bit carby for the early stages of the diet, you can feast on delicious vegetable curry with lots of vegetable side dishes, paneer (Indian cheese) if they do it (a bit carby, but fine for a treat) and really not miss the rice and bread. It's certainly nice to be able to eat a lot and not suffer any after-effects.

Thai and Chinese food can be great, too, but you do have to watch out for sugar and pineapple in some of the sweet and sour dishes.

Middle Eastern food is fine because there are so many delicious vegetable dishes. Avoid the bean and lentil dishes and, instead of hummus, go for creamy tahini sauce or delectable babaganooj (creamy, smoky-flavoured aubergine and tahini dip), crumbly feta and fresh vegetables as a starter. Spanikopita (Greek spinach and feta pie) is fine for vegetarians – eat the lovely filling and leave the filo pastry.

Fast-food places don't offer much for the low-carb vegetarian. If they serve salad you could go for that, avoiding any sweetcorn, pineapple, potato salad and anything that looks as though it might have sugar in it. Pizza is a real no-no, obviously. We can only hope that, as low-carb eating becomes more popular, fast-food outlets will start to broaden their menus.

Buying food when you're travelling is equally difficult: the times I've trekked the length and breadth of a station, tired and hungry, looking for something, anything, that I could eat. They don't even sell little packets of cheese, with or without crackers, any more. It's all sandwiches, croissants, baguettes, Danish pastries … I've sometimes ended up buying the only thing available, a packet of salted peanuts, and learnt to look after myself, as I've been describing, by thinking ahead and taking something with me … perhaps some almonds or Brazil nuts, a piece of cheese, or some protein powder in a plastic screw-top cup, ready to shake with water.

Talking of protein drinks, it's not a bad idea to have one before you go out, if you think the options are going to be limited. That way you can keep up your energy and feel free to enjoy plenty of tasty vegetables, without bothering about the protein.

SOME VEGETARIAN LOW-CARB RESTAURANT DISHES

Starters
- Melon (check no sugar)
- Clear vegetable broth
- Creamy vegetable soups (can be OK but check whether they contain flour or potato)
- Little crunchy fresh salads, with or without cheese (remove any croûtons)
- Tomato and Mozzarella salad with basil and maybe some avocado
- Asparagus
- Avocado
- Artichokes
- Wild or garlic mushrooms (without coatings or batter)
- Fried or grilled Halloumi cheese

▶

Main courses

- Omelettes
- Soufflés (may contain a little flour)
- Egg-based dishes such as Eggs Florentine
- Vegetable and cheese dishes such as Aubergine Parmigiana
- Stir-fry with tofu
- Roasted vegetables with Mozzarella or other cheese
- Aubergines stuffed with cheese, mushrooms, pine nuts
- Red peppers stuffed with cheese, olives, tomatoes
- Quiche (but leave the pastry)

Desserts

- Raspberries or strawberries and cream
- Fresh fruit salad
- Melon

Dining with friends

If eating at restaurants is challenging, dining with friends can be even more so. You'll need all your strength of will and determination to cope. But you can do it, and, as with getting what you want in restaurants, each time you handle the situation with confidence – and realise that your friends don't think any the less of you because you refuse their home-made biscuits or apple pie – it will get easier. Just like the diet, really: the more you do it, the more natural and automatic it becomes. Buffet meals are fine because you can choose exactly what you want, piling up your plate with salad and/or vegetables and bypassing the bread, pasta, rice and potatoes.

It's dinner parties that can be difficult. Telling your host or hostess you're vegetarian is one thing (they can usually handle this, even veganism) but adding that you're also low-carb – somehow that feels like a step too far. I'm all for being honest, though: what you say does depend to some extent on how well you know your host/hostess.

Close friends, I'd tell – as long as I didn't think it would faze them completely – and maybe offer some suggestions as to possible dishes they could make. (Most people have a repertoire of cheese-based dishes, in any case.) Also, lovely vegetable-forget-about-the-protein dishes are great, especially if you make sure you've eaten plenty of protein during the rest of the day.

But what about those people you just can't talk to in advance? These can be the most difficult occasions to handle, especially if your host/hostess has gone to a lot of trouble to make a vegetarian or vegan main course especially for you – and it's a carbohydrate-based one, as they usually are. What you do in these instances depends on the kind of person you are, and the kind of person your host/hostess is, and how strong and confident you have become about asking for what you want.

Some people get around this by saying they're not eating carbs on medical grounds – which is stretching a point (unless you're diabetic or have other sugar-related conditions which the diet is helping) but true, I suppose, in essence. If you're going to say this, then do try to do so in advance. Personally, I think it's best to say something like 'oh, that looks really yummy' and then add 'not *too* big a portion for me ...', turn down potatoes, rice, etc, if you can, or ask for just a tiny bit, but go to town on the vegetables.

When it comes to dessert, if it's berries and cream, you're in luck. Otherwise, if it would be rude and unkind to turn it down, you can plead fullness, because the main course was 'so delicious', and just ask for a tiny bit, unless by that time in the meal you've been able to tell them about your low-carb diet, and can then graciously decline, saying that it looks delicious and you'd love to, but ... If they try to push you, just remain kind but firm.

Even if you do have to eat a meal like this, it really won't do any long-term damage to your diet. The worst that can happen is that you'll put on a pound or two, most of which will be water, since carbohydrate holds water. Or you may feel those carb cravings rearing their ugly heads. You can counter both these problems by having a couple of 'pure' days of protein and vegetables, as in the Carb Cleanse. The most important thing is to stop any possible repercussions occurring, nip them in the bud, put the situation firmly behind you, and move on.

Actually, eating a carby meal occasionally, when there's no alternative, can be quite an eye-opener. You may discover – as do many low-carbers – just how little you enjoy those foods now, and how much better your body feels after you've eaten a low-carb meal.

Cravings, triggers and binges

One of the joys of the Vegetarian Low-Carb Diet is the effect it has on food cravings. Cutting right back on carbs really does break the vicious circle of energy slump, followed by need for quick-energy carbs, followed by quick 'high', followed by energy slump.

In addition to this, being in ketosis (which you probably will be during Phase 1 and 2 of the diet if you're eating less than 45–50g carbs a day) has its own appetite-suppressing effect. So, for most people, food cravings lessen or even disappear completely.

However, you didn't become overweight overnight, and habits aren't easy to break. So don't be surprised if you do feel the old cravings sometimes. It's not the cravings that matter – it's how you deal with them. OK, maybe they used to lead to binge-eating and the 'now I've blown it, I'll start again tomorrow' mentality, but they don't need to any more.

You're a different person. You've changed – or are changing. You are transforming not only your body but also your whole approach to food. To life, even: I do believe that going on this diet can be a life-changing, life-enhancing process of transformation.

POSSIBLE TRIGGERS TO WATCH OUT FOR

- The sight or smell of food, like a TV advert for sweets, or the sight of a plate of chips, say.
- A habitual response, such as always getting the desire to eat a bar of chocolate after visiting your mother-in-law.
- Feeling angry or unloved or unattractive or a failure or afraid of something.
- Or, if you're a woman, it might be pre-menstrual tension (although the Vegetarian Low-Carb Diet with its healthy oils, tofu and other nourishing foods often helps this, as do evening primrose capsules and B vitamins).
- Exposure to pollutants and chemicals such as pesticides, disinfectants, air-fresheners, cosmetics, washing powders and so on can trigger cravings in some people.
- Eating certain foods, which are perfectly fine and healthy for many people, can also be triggers, especially if you're a bit allergic to them. Notice if you usually get a craving after eating a certain food.

Coping with cravings

As a craving is an emotional response – whether induced by erratic blood-sugar levels or by a 'trigger' – it can feel overwhelming. But it needn't be. With practice, and a few strategies (see below), you can learn to cope and, after a while, free yourself from cravings for the most part.

1 Take a pause. Slowly drink some water. If possible, get away from the thing or situation that has triggered the craving.

2 Now ask yourself: 'What is it I *really* want?'

Is it really two dozen cream buns straight away this instant, or is it that you're dead worried about the exam you're taking in a few days' time, or whether your boyfriend is cheating on you, or that you feel fat and ugly, or that you're exhausted by the demands of your two-year-old, or you feel angry that you never have time for yourself ... or any of a million other scenarios?

3 Being self-aware enough to realise what's triggering the craving is one thing; actually stopping it is another. First, if you can, try to think through the problem and work out what would have to be done to improve the situation. Then do it, or at least start the process if that's practical.

4 Next, try one of the following:
  • Go outside and have a little walk
  • Have a relaxing bubble bath
  • Spend some money on a little non-food treat for yourself
  • Put your feet up and read a book or magazine
  • Do a crossword
  • Phone a friend
  • Listen to some music that always puts you in a good mood
  • Watch a video
  • Stroke and cuddle the cat
  • Go for a swim

It's not a bad idea to keep a list like this somewhere handy and promise yourself you'll refer to it before giving in to your craving.

5 If all else fails ... give in.

Yes, give in to your craving. BUT – and this is the crucial bit – give in with low-carb foods. Give yourself permission to eat as much as you want, for an hour, an evening, a day even, if it's one of those days when you wake up hungry and keep on wanting to eat all day. (Though, I promise you, they'll be far, far fewer once you've been low-carbing for a bit.)

Take a moment to identify what it is about the food you're *really* wanting. Is it something crisp, crunchy, salty? Or sweet and crunchy, like breakfast cereal, crisp biscuits, or nut brittle? Or hot, savoury and soothing, like mashed potatoes or home-made potato soup? Or sweet, rich and creamy, like ice-cream or a thick, icy milk shake? Or is it 'stodge' you're after, like bread with lots of butter? Or maybe it's cake, fruit pie or just good old chips? All of these desires can be satisfied with low-carb alternatives (see below).

Low-carb alternatives

The following is a quick guide to low-carb alternatives. An increasing number of manufactured low-carb foods are coming on to the market (see p. 319, for some specialist stockists). To be honest, apart from the odd low-carb bar, I haven't tried any of them myself. I much prefer making my own food at home – it's far, far cheaper and I like to know what's in it. In fact, a number of dieters in the US have found some manufactured low-carb foods more of a hindrance than a help (see p. 54).

While the following home-made low-carb alternatives may not taste quite the same as the foods they're replacing, they do generally 'hit the spot'. And it's so lovely to be able to indulge shamelessly, knowing that what you're eating won't be doing too much damage to your health or your weight.

It's important to make sure you have these foods readily available (stashed in the cupboard, or freezer if necessary) so that when you just have to grab the nearest something, it's a low-carb something. Of course, it helps if you no longer keep stocks of carby foods but that's probably only an option if you live on your own.

When you fancy some cereal ...

Crunchy breakfast cereal
You could try a crunchy home-made mix of flaked almonds and ground flax seeds (linseeds), or the Crunchy Granola recipe on p. 148. You can buy various low-carb breakfast cereals from low-carb

suppliers but I haven't tried any myself. If breakfast cereal is a comfort food for you, it could be worth finding out what's available so you're prepared for a craving. Some people mix low-carb 'puffed wheat' cereal with ordinary puffed wheat cereal, which is fairly low in carbs. Have it with lots of soya milk or cream and whatever low-carb sweetener you like to use.

Hot breakfast cereal

If it's comforting hot cereal you crave, you can make Sara's Hot Cereal (see p. 149), a very satisfying kind of porridge using ground almonds, which you could top with cream, or you can try a delicious Ricotta 'Rice' Pudding (see p. 290).

When you fancy a snack ...

Bread

If it's bread you want, you'll need to be prepared, with some home-made Low-Carb Bread (p. 294), sliced and in the freezer. It thaws very quickly – you can toast it straight from frozen. Or you could make the Instant Microwave Low-Carb Bread (see p. 293), which is a bit more 'cakey', but very quick. I love all the bread recipes I've given in this book. They don't taste quite like 'normal' bread, but I think they're good in their own right. You can buy low-carb bread from some of the specialist shops listed in the back of this book (see p. 319) but, again, I haven't tried any of them. You could also buy some low-carb jam to have on your bread or toast or you could have it with lashings of butter …

Crisps or tortilla chips

Make some Cheese Crisps (see p. 205) or cut firm tofu into paper-thin slices – as thin as you can without tearing – and fry them in olive oil on both sides until crisp and golden. Sprinkle with salt and serve with lots of Mayonnaise (see p. 187), soured cream or Avocado Dip (see p. 200).

Crackers

You can easily make some great low-carb crackers from the recipe on p. 296. Eat them with butter and cheese if that's what you're craving.

When you fancy something hot and filling ...

Pasta

Use soya noodles if you can – they're sometimes found in the chill cabinet in Asian shops – or low-carb pasta (available from specialist shops, see p. 319). Soya-based pasta is good because it supplies protein. Spaghetti squash is also a delicious substitute, as are courgette and cabbage 'pasta' dishes (see pp. 229–39).

Chips/French fries

Turnip Chips (see p. 264) look a bit like potato chips and are great for dipping into Easy Tomato Ketchup (see p. 189). I love them, but I can't pretend they taste like chips and they never get really crisp. If you want them crisp, try Roasted Cauliflower (see p. 267) – don't laugh – which does get crisp round the edges and is great for dipping into Mayonnaise (see p. 187).

Roast potatoes

Try Roasted Cauliflower (see p. 267) or Turnip Roast Potatoes (see p. 264). You can also roast kohlrabi, which has a lovely delicate flavour, and salsify, if you can find it.

Mashed potatoes

You can make glorious, light, fluffy 'mashed potatoes' (see Cauliflower Mash on p. 260) by whizzing cooked cauliflower, turnips or celeriac with butter or olive oil, seasoning and some double cream (or soya cream). Some people whiz in some cream cheese or tofu, too, to give it more body. It's not as starchy as mashed potatoes, of course, but I think it's pretty good.

When you fancy something sweet ...

Something crisp, sweet and chocolaty

Make a batch of Chocolate Almond Bark (see p. 306). It's very quick to do and one of my favourites. You can even make it taste like chocolate mint crisps if you add a drop or two of peppermint oil.

Chunky, chewy chocolate bars

Try chocolate low-carb bars.

Sweet biscuits

Buy ready-made, low-carb biscuits from a specialist store or make your own from the recipes in the recipe section (see pp. 299–309).

Fruit pie

Try the Rhubarb Crumble recipe (see p. 284) or Blueberry Pie (see p. 286), served with plenty of cream or soya cream.

Jelly

You can make a wonderful Red Fruit Jelly (see p. 274), which contains virtually no carbs at all.

When you fancy something rich and creamy ...

Milk shakes

Whiz frozen strawberries or raspberries, straight from the freezer, with stevia or low-carb sweetening to taste, unsweetened soya milk and a dash of double cream if you like, to make a thick Creamy Berry Smoothie (see p. 138).

Ice-cream

Make instant Raspberry Ice-Cream (see p. 277) in the same way as the smoothie, above, but use more frozen fruit so you get a thicker mixture.

Flavoured yogurt

Low-carb live yogurt – thick Greek, if you like it creamy, with your choice of stevia or low-carb sweetener and flavouring stirred in. You can buy a wide range of different flavouring essences in the baking department of large supermarkets. Or make a batch of Creamy Berry 'Yogurt' (see p. 275).

Rich creamy dessert

Whip some double cream until thick, then fold in stevia or low-carb sweetener and flavouring to taste; or some fresh berries, ground almonds – whatever low-carb extras you fancy. Or try sweetening canned, unsweetened rhubarb with a little stevia and serving with lots of whipped double cream.

Getting back on the diet

What if none of this works and you eat the two dozen cream buns and a zillion other things as well?

Don't give yourself stick. It's not the end of the world. Tomorrow is another day, as they say, and you can get right back on the Carb Cleanse, and repair the damage very quickly. Get something really positive out of the experience, if you can, by recognising what triggered your craving, so that you can avoid or deal with the situation if it recurs.

First of all, you need to know that it takes about 48 hours on the Carb Cleanse to get rid of the stored sugar in your body and to make it switch from carb-burning to fat-burning. During this first 48 hours, whether you're just starting the diet for the first time, or you have had a bit of a lapse and are going back to the Carb Cleanse to get on track again, you may well have strong cravings for the carbs you're cutting back on.

Forewarned is forearmed, so if you know that this is likely to happen, you can prepare. Try to do the Carb Cleanse when you'll be least tempted by carbohydrates around you, and pick a time when you're not likely to be thinking much about food. This might be when you're very busy with work, or over a weekend, perhaps, when you can plan a lot of activities that will stop you focusing on any cravings.

Having said that, if you feel weak and hungry all the time, or even depressed, as some people do during these first two or three days on the diet, my advice is to feel free to eat as much of the 'allowed' foods as you want. Just eat, particularly, the proteins: eggs, cheese and tofu. Hard-boiled eggs or Devilled Eggs (see p. 193) are wonderfully filling.

Although cheese is limited to about 115g (4oz) during the diet, if it helps you to get through this stage, please feel free to eat more. Tofu can be very satisfying, too: try slicing firm tofu as thinly as you can (2–3mm/⅟₁₆–⅛in), shallow-frying the strips in olive oil then serving them with Mayonnaise (see p. 187) or Avocado Dip (see p. 200). This is a great substitute for crisps and tortillas.

Once you're past the first couple of days and are getting into low-carb habits again and feeling calmer and more energised, you'll be able to cut back your food and carbs again naturally and get on with the diet.

There are a few people who find that they really can't drop to 20g carbs a day 'just like that': they need to decrease their carbs more slowly, perhaps starting at, say 50–60g on the first day, then dropping to 40g and so on, until they reach 20g – or 30g, if 20g is too low. Some people, like Sara, find this rehabilitation process quite difficult.

She says: 'I'm one of those people who have a hard time getting into ketosis. I get headaches, fatigue, sometimes muscle pain. So when I binge and then drop back down I have to be careful about that and sometimes I have to lower my carb count gradually. Other times it's not bad and I just ride it out. Either way, I know that in 48 hours I'm going to be feeling great again.'

One way of easing yourself gently back into low-carb eating again after you've lapsed, for whatever reason, is simply to concentrate, at first, on increasing the protein you eat at every meal and snack. Just try adding extra protein for a day or two without changing anything else. Then, when you've adapted to that, add extra vegetables or salad at every meal, too.

Try to eat the protein and vegetables or salad *before* you eat any carbohydrate you might be having. And each day increase the amount of protein and vegetables until you can drop the carbs. Then you can start carb-counting again and, before you know it, you'll be in ketosis, back on track and feeling great.

Most people go into ketosis if they eat less than 50g carbs a day, although everyone is different, so it's best not to generalise. And once ketosis happens, then even for those who've got there slowly, the same benefits apply. As one low-carb veggy dieter says: 'When I do finally get into ketosis, it's wonderful. I feel great, I'm not hungry all the time, I go whole hours without even THINKING about food. For me, that's very liberating, quite apart from the joy of the weight loss part.'

As the diet progresses, and you add in more carbs, ketosis will gradually tail off. Your body will still be burning fat, and your insulin levels will remain steady. But you won't get the natural appetite-suppressant effect of ketosis and old binge habits may recur.

That's why it's important to stay on the diet long enough for it to change your eating habits and emotional responses to food. The golden rules of having regular meals, not going more than six waking hours without eating, and concentrating on getting enough protein and healthy fat will stand you in good stead. They will ensure that you satisfy your appetite and stabilise your blood-sugar level.

Dealing with a plateau

Oh, the pain of the plateau. Is there a dieter anywhere who doesn't know it? One minute you're doing fine, losing weight steadily, even if it's not coming off *quite* as fast as you'd like. Then suddenly you get stuck. One week passes, then another – and maybe another, or even more, and that pesky needle on the scale budges not one jot. Or it may even threaten to move upwards. So, what to do?

First, ask yourself whether you've already reached a weight that's good for you

Sometimes dieters try to get thinner than their bodies really want to go. It may be that you've reached a healthy weight for you, even if it's not quite your idea of the 'ideal' weight.

Check whether you're gaining muscle as fast as you're losing fat

Many low-carb dieters reach a point where they stop losing weight for a while but continue to slim down. This is because the combination of exercise and the healthy diet are building muscle, which is more compact than fat. So you weigh the same, or even a shade more, but look leaner and firmer and, perhaps the most crucial test of all, your clothes fit better. If this is the case, then just keep doing what you're doing – not forgetting that all-important exercise – and you'll soon break through the plateau.

Are you doing enough exercise?

Many people find that, as they increase the exercise, they decrease the weight. So, burn, burn, burn ... Doing more exercise will increase muscle which may initially make matters worse, weight-wise, but, as I've explained above, you'll actually be thinner – and very soon the scale will start telling you the same thing as your waistbands.

Double-check your diet

Are you counting your carbs accurately, or have you got a bit careless? Are you reading packet labels carefully? Are you eating something with 'hidden carbs' that you weren't eating before? Cough sweets, chewable vitamins, some medicines, for instance, can contain quite a bit of sugar. Or is there a particular food, which, though healthy in itself, is causing your weight to stall? Dairy and wheat products, for instance, can have this effect on some people. Cut back on any foods that you think could be causing the problem and see what happens.

Are you still eating enough fat, protein and calories?

It might be helpful to 'retrace your steps' for a week or two and go back to eating as you did in the Carb Cleanse – partly to remind you of the importance of eating regularly, not going more than six waking hours without food, and getting enough fat and protein.

Are you taking in too many calories?

While you need to make sure you eat enough calories – otherwise your body may go into 'starvation mode' and cling on to the weight for survival – it's also important to make sure you're not eating excessive calories. Although, as I explained in Chapter 1, you can eat more calories on the Vegetarian Low-Carb Diet (see p. 13), if you exceed your body's needs, it will still store the rest as fat. Even this diet can't defy the laws of thermodynamics – alas! So, just be aware of this and, if you're eating very calorific foods (lots of nuts, or cream, for instance), cut back on them a bit and see what happens.

Are you taking your vitamins?

Sometimes the body clings to weight because it's lacking some nutrient – another survival technique. So make sure you're still taking your multivitamin, and consider adding some chromium. A daily dose of 400–600 micrograms of chromium picolinate or chromium polynicotinate, spread evenly throughout the day, with meals, can help carb-burning. L-carnitine can be helpful, too. The usual dose is 1000–3000 milligrams a day. (This is just as good for weight loss as the more expensive Acetyl-L-carnitine, which helps brain power, promotes longevity and also lifts your spirits – worth its weight in gold, in my book, though not essential. Q10 is another supplement that is also very worthwhile for the 'feel good' factor it can bring.)

Is the problem emotional or psychological?

This is a little beyond the scope of this book, but sometimes emotional or psychological factors can hinder weight loss. Fear of success, or of getting into a relationship once they're slim, for instance, can make people consciously or unconsciously stall their weight loss. If you think this might be true for you, a few sessions with a good counsellor could be very helpful.

Six secrets of staying slim for ever

Finally, to help you keep your lovely lean, strong, healthy body for ever, here are Six Secrets of Staying Slim:

1. Keep to your carb level – you will certainly know what that is by now.

2. Resolve right now that you will weigh yourself once a week, and that you won't go more than 5lb above your goal weight without taking action. That means going back on the Carb Cleanse for a few days, a week, or however long it takes to get back to your goal weight.

3. Watch out for your trigger foods and situations and be prepared (see the tips on pp. 114–7).

4. Take your vitamins.

5. Keep up your exercise.

6. Enjoy your meals and have fun experimenting with different ingredients, flavours and foods.

The Recipes

INTRODUCTION

'It's all about the food,' they say about low-carb dieting, and it's true. The food is great. And that, apart from the fact that you lose weight well and feel good, is why so many people find this is the one diet they can stick to. You may have to be adaptable and change your mind-set on some foods, but you know that you can always look forward to a good meal. What's more, the chances are it's a meal which other people are happy to eat, too – and you can't say that of many diets.

The food doesn't have to be complicated and time-consuming to prepare, either. In fact you can eat very simply, with the minimum of cooking, if you wish. Crunchy salads with lovely cheeses, buttery omelettes, crisply fried tofu dipped in mayonnaise, steamed or stir-fried vegetables with grated cheese or spicy tofu, vegetarian sausages with 'mash', sweet berries with cream … You can certainly do this diet successfully – and stay on it – while spending the minimum of time in the kitchen, just concentrating on lovely fresh produce … so easy, so delicious, so healthy.

However, if you want to spend a little more time in the kitchen, there are hundreds of wonderful things you can make and they really will add interest and variety, especially when you've been on the diet for some time. I have found it rewarding and fun to experiment with low-carb cooking – it's amazing what you can do. Some of the results of my experiments follow: I hope you'll enjoy them.

The recipes are arranged in the following sections:

Drinks, Shakes and Smoothies: This section has plenty of tips on how to make nutritious drinks, ranging from a morning Energy Shake to a soothing Low-Carb Hot Chocolate for the evening.

Breakfast Dishes: Having got this far in the book, I'm sure you've realised that breakfast can be pretty well anything you fancy – eggs, cheese, tofu, baked dishes, ice-cream – as long as it's rich in protein and low in carbs. For this reason, you can find things to eat for breakfast in every recipe section. But here I've focused first on breakfast cereals, hot and cold, and how to make yogurt and soya milk. If you fancy a more substantial cooked breakfast, there are all sorts of options, including omelettes, Scrambled Eggs on a Mushroom, or Flaky Smoked Tofu.

Quick Lunches and Snacks: For lunch, there are lots of easy soups, like Comforting Cauliflower and a tasty Tomato Cheddar Soup. You'll also find your favourite salads, such as Greek, Caesar, Niçoise, and Hot Goat's Cheese, which you can serve with Vinaigrette, Mayonnaise, and other dressings and sauces. And when you feel peckish at any time of day, there are plenty of easy, creamy dips, from Avocado Dip to Sesame and Tofu Hummus, to eat with savoury snacks like Cheese Crisps and Crunchy Tofu Sticks.

Main Meals: This section starts with quick stir-fries and grills, from Oriental-style dishes to Cheesy Portobello 'Steaks' and Low-Carb Vegeburgers. Then there are some great curries, including Thai Coconut Curry, and Tandoori Tofu. There are also low-carb alternatives for perhaps the most popular stove-top dish of all, pasta, with recipes for Cabbage Tagliatelle with Red Pepper and Artichoke Hearts and Courgette Ribbon Pasta with Mushroom Cream Sauce, among others. When you fancy something warming, there are all sorts of baked dishes, from wonderful Low-Carb Pizza to the delicious layered aubergine dish, Parmigiana, and Nut Roast with Lemon Sauce. Vegetables and side dishes include low-carb favourites such as Cauliflower Mash (which I now like better than ordinary mash), Turnip Roast Potatoes, Roasted Ratatouille and Spiced Spinach.

Puddings: This section has some refreshing sorbets and a clear jelly, as well as several ices, creams and mousses. If you feel like finishing your meal with something hot, there's low-carb Ricotta 'Rice' Pudding, a delicious Rhubarb Crumble and some Little Egg Custards.

Baked Treats and Sweets: Here you'll find several types of low-carb bread, some crisp Almond Crackers, a Baked Lemon Cheesecake, Nut Muffins, gooey Chocolate Brownies, and Almond Chocolate Bark, which breaks with a delightful 'snap'.

Making Life Easy in the Kitchen

I'm all for making life as easy as you can for yourself. A major challenge for any dieter is having to cook meals when you're tired and hungry, particularly if this means cooking high-carb foods for other people. The way to cope with this is to think ahead, so that you know what you're going to make, and you have the ingredients you need.

Try to make a habit of sitting down once a week and thinking about the next seven days. Will there be times when you'll be out-and-about and may be too busy to eat? Will there be times when the people around you may be eating things like pizza or chips, which might tempt you if you don't have your own alternatives easily available?

Decide what you're going to eat on these occasions, as well as for the rest of the week's meals, perhaps using the fortnight of menus (see pp. 73–86) as a basis, and the Ideas for Meals that appear at the beginning of each recipe section. Check out the recipes you want to try, then make a shopping list (see pp. 67–71).

Try to do all your shopping, or as much of it as you can, in one go. Then set aside an evening, or half a day at the weekend, to do your preparations for the next seven days. This will make life so much easier during the week. Here's what to do:

- Wash all the vegetables. Then peel and chop the robust ones (like turnip and cauliflower) and put them into sealed plastic containers in the fridge.

- Rather than buy expensive pre-washed packs of salad (see p. 169), I make up my own mix of salad leaves. I buy a variety of whole lettuces – perhaps a couple of red-leaf ones, an iceberg, a couple of Romaine, a couple of Little Gem, a bunch or two of watercress or rocket (yes, whole bunches, if I can get them) or whatever looks crisp and fresh. After washing them all thoroughly, I shake them dry, then layer them with kitchen paper in large plastic lidded boxes and store them in the fridge. (Layering with kitchen paper works brilliantly for herbs such as basil, too – it's the best way to ensure you've got fresh herbs readily available, short of living on a Greek island with a basil plant growing in the sunshine by your back door.)

- Hard-boil a large batch of eggs – maybe a dozen – for salad meals and quick snacks. Simply put the eggs into a large saucepan, cover with cold water, add 1 tablespoon malt vinegar (the cheapest stuff), 1 teaspoon salt and bring to the boil. Then remove the pan from the heat, cover, and leave for 20 minutes. Drain, plunge the eggs into cold water to cool them quickly, and store in the fridge until required. The shells will slip off like silk.

- If you like bottled salad dressing, make up a batch of Vinaigrette (see p. 185), or make sure you've added salad dressing to your shopping list, and that you get one that's carb-free, or virtually carb-free.

- Now make one or two main dishes. I recommend a batch of Spinach 'Bread' (see p. 159), because it's so versatile and useful. Some Oven-Baked Mushroom Frittata (see p. 155) is wonderful to have in the fridge for quick breakfasts and lunches, and Low-Carb Pizza (see p. 255) is a lifesaver because you can use it straight from the freezer.

- A vegetable casserole is another useful dish to make up in quantity – just follow the Vegetable Soup recipe on p. 168, adding any vegetables that are in season. It's quick to heat up and you can add a variety of extras when you serve it (such as tofu chunks for you, and meat protein or carby additions such as sweetcorn or couscous for non-dieting family members) – hopefully pleasing different tastes.

- If you have the time, a low-carb Nut Roast (see p. 249) is useful to have in the freezer, frozen in slices that you can remove one at a time. Some home-made Low-Carb Bread (see p. 294) is also great, again, sliced before freezing, for easy use.

Equipment

There are a few pieces of equipment which are really helpful for this kind of cooking. Firstly, you'll need some accurate electronic scales. These do not have to do anything other than give you the weight of the ingredients, so you can get the cheapest type – I like the ones which can switch from imperial to metric.

If you're going to do much cooking, a good food processor will save you hours. You can make most of the recipes – more slowly – without a food processor, but there are one or two for which it's essential. I would also class a robust electric coffee-grinder as pretty much a necessity, for grinding up golden flax seeds and also for powdering almonds to a flour which is used in many recipes.

Finally, a new acquisition for me, but one that is getting a lot of use, is a stick blender. Mine has both a chopping and a whisking attachment and is fabulous for whizzing up shakes, smoothies, instant ice-cream and a million other things. I don't know how I ever managed without one. You can also use it straight in the pan to liquidise a soup or sauce, which is handy if you're making a small quantity.

Something else which I seem to use quite a bit for low-carb cookery is non-stick baking paper, so it's a good idea to get some of that, especially if you're going to do any baking.

Quick Diet Re-Cap

Remember, the Vegetarian Low-Carb Diet has three simple principles: cut carbs, add fat, boost protein.

The diet has three phases. In Phase 1, the Carb Cleanse, carbs are cut to 20g a day. In Phase 2, Continued Weight Loss, the daily carbs can be anything from 20g to 60g a day – enough to allow for a weekly weight loss of 1–2lb. Finally, in Phase 3, Maintenance, the daily carbs are increased to a level which keeps your weight steady. (For more about all of this, see pp. 18–45 and 94–106.)

You need to count the carbs in everything – in your protein foods as well as in the salads and vegetables you eat. As the diet progresses, you'll find this gets really easy and automatic and you'll probably be able to eat as much salad and as many low-carb vegetables as you want, without bothering to count. But when you first start the diet, it's a good idea to make a note of your carbs each day.

When reading labels on packets, you can usually subtract the fibre from the carbs, to get the 'net' or 'usable' carbs (as explained on p. 24). I say 'usually' because sometimes the carbs given have already had the fibre taken off – so you need to be a little wary. All the carb counts given in this book are 'usable' carbs: the fibre has already been subtracted.

Throughout the diet, you need to eat at least 60g protein a day – a shade more, maybe 70g, if you're a man. This is not high protein; it's adequate protein – what you need to be healthy.

Fat is fine as long as it's healthy fat – organic butter or cream, extra-virgin olive oil, coconut oil – but avoid margarine, shortening, hydrogenated or partly hydrogenated fat, harmful 'trans' fats (produced when plant oils are partially hardened), or products containing them.

For full details of how to do the diet, see Chapters 1 to 7 of this book and refer back to the 12 Golden Rules for Success (see pp. 42–5).

Ingredients

Nearly all the ingredients used in the recipes are easily available. For more about them, see Chapter 2 in the Diet section of this book. There are a few unusual ingredients that you may need to send away for – but you can do the Vegetarian Low-Carb Diet perfectly well without them. You'll find details of these less usual items under Sources and Stockists (see p. 319).

Using the Recipes

Recipes are given in metric and imperial measurements. As always, it's best to stick to one or the other throughout the recipe, though I've done my best to keep the equivalents as close as possible.

For each recipe, I've listed the phase or phases of the diet for which it is most suitable. Preparation and cooking times are given, as well as the grams of protein and carbs in the recipe. Vegan recipes are indicated with a 'V' symbol.

For non-vegan recipes, I've given vegan alternatives whenever possible, either in the list of ingredients or, if a slightly different method is needed, as a Vegan Variation, at the end of the recipe. Make sure that any vegan replacements for ingredients (such as vegan cheese or fake meats) are as low in carbs as possible, and adjust the carb count of the recipe a little if necessary.

Drinks, Shakes and Smoothies

Shakes and smoothies are easy to make, and great any time – with a meal for extra protein, instead of a meal, or between meals as an energy-booster. Just put your ingredients into a blender, or into the goblet that comes with a stick blender, or even into a plastic screw-top cup, and whiz, blend or shake until thick, smooth and frothy. Then drink.

For a protein-rich shake, start with 1–2 scoops protein powder (either whey powder or soya protein isolate powder). Then add your choice from the following:

Liquid: Bought, unsweetened, or Home-Made Soya Milk (see p. 145), which can be chocolate- or vanilla-flavoured as long as it's unsweetened; plain yogurt, kefir or Home-Made Soya Yogurt (see p. 147); black coffee; strong, carb-free herbal tea such as mint, ginger or a fruit-flavoured tea, or just plain water.

Enrichments: These can be as simple as 1–3 teaspoons flaxseed oil, a tablespoonful of cream or soya cream, a chunk of tofu, a spoonful of cream cheese, or a tablespoonful of peanut or other nut butter.

Some of these increase the protein – soya milk, tofu and peanut butter whizzed together make a beautiful, creamy, protein-rich shake without any protein powder, and taste delicious. You can also add ground almonds to a shake, and almond butter is lovely, too, though expensive.

Fruit and vegetables: If you add raspberries, strawberries or blueberries straight from the freezer, they give a lovely ice-creamy texture. Canned pumpkin, which you can sometimes buy in the UK in large supermarkets, has the same effect. Remember to count the carbs when adding these ingredients. Although you don't need very much, the carbs do add up.

Flavourings: Cocoa powder, grated orange or lemon rind, pure vanilla, almond or lemon extract (try lemon extract or some grated lemon rind and some cream cheese in the mix for a cheesecake-flavoured shake); fresh mint, and any spices you fancy – cinnamon, ginger, allspice, mixed spice, grated nutmeg, a pinch of ground cloves ... A very tiny pinch of salt can also sometimes bring out the flavours but be careful not to overdo it.

Sweetenings: Add these at the end, because many of the ingredients taste sweet and you may be surprised at how little extra you need to add. (For more about choice of sweetener, see p. 35–8.)

CREAMY BERRY SMOOTHIE

Phases 2/3 **Ⓥ**
Preparation: 2–3 minutes

SERVES 1

55g (2oz) frozen summer fruits (e.g. raspberries, strawberries, blueberries)

150ml (5fl oz) water

2 scoops micro-filtered whey powder or soya protein isolate

55g (2oz) firm tofu (optional – if you like it thicker)

1 tablespoon whipping cream or soya cream

stevia or Splenda tablets to taste

1. Put the ingredients into a blender, food processor or the goblet that comes with a stick blender, and whiz together, for about 15 seconds, until blended.

2. Sweeten to taste with stevia or Splenda. Add 0.5 carbs per teaspoon if using powdered Splenda, or avoid this by using the tablets (dissolved in a little water before adding).

3. Drink immediately.

> 5g carbs and 52g protein

CHOCOLATE ENERGY SHAKE

Phases 1/2/3 Ⓥ
Preparation: 2–3 minutes

You can use unsweetened soya milk instead of water for this shake.

SERVES 1
1 scoop non-GMO soya isolate powder

1 teaspoon cocoa powder

1 level tablespoon unsweetened peanut butter

200ml (7fl oz) water

Put the ingredients into a blender, food processor or the goblet that comes with a stick blender, and whiz until blended and frothy, adding more water if you wish.

> 2.6g carbs and 30g protein

ENERGY SHAKE

Phases 1/2/3 Ⓥ
Preparation: 2–3 minutes

You can use unsweetened soya milk instead of water for this shake, and you can add cream, tofu, cream cheese, vanilla, spices or any other flavourings you fancy. Just remember to add any 'carby' additions to your total carb count.

SERVES 1
1 scoop non-GMO soya isolate powder

1 level tablespoon unsweetened peanut butter

200ml (7fl oz) water

Put the ingredients into a blender, food processor or the goblet that comes with a stick blender, and whiz until blended and frothy, adding more water if you wish.

> 2g carbs and 30g protein

Variation:

This shake is also delicious made with roasted almond butter.

PEANUT SMOOTHIE

Phases 1/2/3 Ⓥ
Preparation: 2–3 minutes

This is creamy and rich-tasting, satisfying and filling. It's also good made with almond butter.

SERVES 1
200ml (7fl oz) unsweetened soya milk, bought or home-made
   (see p. 145)
2 tablespoons unsweetened peanut butter
1 tablespoon dairy or soya cream
1 teaspoon cocoa powder (optional)
1 teaspoon real vanilla extract (optional)

1. Put the ingredients into a blender, food processor or the goblet that comes with a stick blender, and whiz until blended and frothy, adding more water if you wish.

2. Taste and add sweetener of your choice if needed: it's quite sweet as it is.

> 6.3g carbs and 17.2g protein

CHOCOLATE TOFU SMOOTHIE

Phases 1/2/3 Ⓥ
Preparation: 2–3 minutes

SERVES 1
55g (2oz) firm tofu
150–200ml (5–7fl oz) soya milk, bought or home-made (see p. 145)
2 teaspoons cocoa powder
2 level teaspoons peanut butter
2 tablespoons whipping or soya cream
stevia or Splenda tablets to taste

1. Put the ingredients into a blender, food processor or the goblet that comes with a stick blender, and whiz together until blended. Drink immediately.

> 5g carbs and 14g protein

LOW-CARB HOT CHOCOLATE

Phases 1/2/3 Ⓥ
Preparation: 2–3 minutes

This makes a nice, soothing, protein-rich drink.

SERVES 1
2 teaspoons cocoa powder
stevia to taste or 1–2 Splenda tablets
250ml (9fl oz) unsweetened soya milk, bought or home-made
    (see p. 145)
a little double, whipping or soya cream to taste (optional)

1. Put the cocoa and stevia or Splenda tablets into a mug. Heat the soya milk, add to the mug and stir well. Add a little cream if you like, either mixed in or whipped on top. (Double cream is 0.5g carbs per tablespoonful.)

> 2g carbs and 10.3g protein (without cream)

MOCK MARGARITA

Phases 1/2/3 Ⓥ
Preparation: 2–3 minutes

This refreshing drink doesn't contain any alcohol, but may hit the spot nevertheless. Flavoured waters can be an excellent substitute for sugary or caffeinated soft drinks. Just check the label for carbs, and avoid aspartame, which can stall weight loss.

SERVES 1
1 lime
1–2 good sprigs fresh mint
ice
200ml (7fl oz) sugar-free lime- and lemon-flavoured sparkling water, chilled

1. Halve the lime, squeeze out the juice and put into a glass. Bruise the rinds and the mint sprigs with the end of a wooden spoon to help release the oils. Add the rinds and mint sprigs to the glass, along with some ice, then pour in the flavoured water and drink at once.

> 1g carbs and 0g protein

Breakfast Dishes

Having a good breakfast really can set you up, energy-wise, for the rest of the day, and is one of the fundamentals of the Vegetarian Low-Carb Diet. Please don't skip breakfast. And, whatever you eat, make sure it's packed with protein – at least 20g. When you start doing this, you'll soon notice the difference.

If mornings are a rush for you, try to plan ahead. A good breakfast can be simple; it can be eaten on the run, it can be prepared when you get to work: just make sure you have it.

The recipes in this section are for cereals and cooked breakfasts, but there are good breakfast choices throughout this book, from shakes and smoothies, to cheese and egg dishes, to main course bakes, to puddings, and low-carb breads and cakes. There's plenty of choose from. Here are some suggestions:

- A protein-rich shake or smoothie – if necessary, keep some whey powder or soya protein isolate powder at work and whiz up a shake when you arrive, or carry some with you in a plastic screw-top cup, ready to shake with water. This is great when you're out and about and it may be hard to find a low-carb, protein-rich meal.

- Plain, unsweetened soya milk yogurt (bought or home-made, see p. 147) or Greek yogurt, topped with whole or ground flax seeds (linseeds), chopped almonds, hazelnuts, walnuts or pumpkin seeds.

- A piece of cheese, a hard-boiled egg and a handful of almonds.

- Some Marinated Tofu (see p. 219). Pack into a container for breakfast-on-the-run.

- A two- or three-egg omelette filled with a little grated cheese, fried mushrooms or chopped herbs. Can be made the night before, packed and eaten cold – it's surprisingly good.

- A vegetarian/vegan cooked breakfast, including any of the following: vegetarian sausages, vegetarian fake bacon, or smoked tofu (cut thinly and fried until crisp), tomatoes, mushrooms, fried eggs ... Choose your vegetarian sausages and bacon carefully because the carb content varies greatly. There are some very low-carb ones and I hope more will soon become available.

- Spinach 'Bread' (see p. 159), spread with cream cheese, or chopped hard-boiled eggs and mayonnaise, or slices of cheese or peanut butter, to make a green 'sandwich'. You really have to try this to understand how good it is.

- Low-carb bread, bought or home-made (see p. 294), plain or toasted, with peanut butter, perhaps made into a sandwich for easy carrying.

- Crunchy Granola (see p. 148), with soya cream or soya yogurt, bought or home-made (see p. 147).

- For 'Sara's Hot Cereal' (see p. 149), make up the 'dry' mix and keep it at work if you like. Then just add boiling water, mix and eat for a great start to the day.

- Home-Made Nut Muffins (see p. 302).

- A portion of your previous evening's meal to heat up for a quick and savoury breakfast.

- A fruity tofu 'whiz' or fool, light and protein-packed, rather like a thick fruit yogurt (see p. 280).

HOME-MADE SOYA MILK

Phases 1/2/3
Preparation: 20 minutes (plus overnight soaking)
Cooking: 30 minutes

Sara Byk, whose inspiring story appears on p. 59, is not only a very successful low-carber, she also makes all her own soya milk for herself and her family. This recipe is based on her method and I'm indebted to her for sharing it.

MAKES 1 LITRE (1¾ PINTS)
350g (12oz) dried yellow soya beans
1.3 litres (2¼ pints) water, plus extra for soaking and boiling
2 teaspoons bicarbonate of soda

Optional flavourings:
chunk of raw fresh ginger root
½ vanilla pod

1. Cover the beans with their height again in cold water and soak overnight, or for at least 8 hours.

2. Bring a large saucepan of water to the boil – and also put the kettle on, for more. It really speeds up this recipe if you have plenty of boiling water available.

3. Drain the beans into a colander, rinse under the cold tap, then put them into the pan of boiling water, add 1 teaspoon of bicarb, bring back to the boil, and simmer, uncovered, for 5 minutes.

4. Drain the beans into the colander again, discarding all the water. Rinse the beans under the tap, put back into the pan with boiling water from the kettle, to cover, and 1 teaspoon bicarb. Bring to the boil, and simmer, uncovered, for 5 minutes.

5. Drain the beans into a colander again, as before, and rinse under the tap.

6. Put the beans back into the saucepan, this time with the quantity of water given in the ingredients, and either of the additional flavourings if you want to use them. (They're both nice variations, but this milk also tastes good without additional flavouring.) Bring to the boil and simmer for 5 minutes. Then remove from the heat and allow to cool.

7. Using a food processor or stick blender, purée the beans thoroughly, then strain through a sieve lined with a piece of scalded muslin, pressing the muslin with your hands to wring out the last few drops.

8. The result will be the most beautiful, creamy soya milk. Keep in the fridge. You could also make your own tofu from this milk – but that's probably something for another book!

0.4g carbs and 3.7g protein per 100ml (3½fl oz)

HOME-MADE SOYA YOGURT

Phase 1/2/3
Preparation: 15 minutes / Cooking: 10–15 minutes

It's really easy to make your own soya yogurt – and it can also be the basis of a wonderful Vegan Cream Cheese (see p. 199). Incidentally, if you use live Greek yogurt as a 'starter', as I do, the first batch of yogurt will not be totally vegan. However, you can save a couple of teaspoonfuls to start your next batch, which will be vegan.

You need a warm place in which to incubate the yogurt. You can create this by heating the oven to 200°C (400°F) Gas Mark 6 and then turning it off. Or you could wrap the jars in a warm towel and put them by a radiator. My own 'Heath Robinson' method is to fill a hot water bottle with boiling water and put into an insulated box – the kind used to keep food hot or cold. I put some pieces of polystyrene packing and towels on top, then the jars of yogurt, then more towelling and close the lid. I have perfect yogurt after 6–8 hours.

MAKES 1 LITRE (1¾ PINTS)
1 litre (1¾ pints) unsweetened organic soya milk, bought or home-made (see p. 145)
1–2 teaspoons plain live yogurt (I use live Greek yogurt)

1. You will need three clean 450g (1lb) jam or honey jars with screw-top lids. Fill the jars with boiling water from the kettle, pour some boiling water over the lids, too, and set aside to sterilise.

2. Put the milk into a saucepan and bring to the boil, then remove from the heat and leave until it is tepid (slightly warm to the touch).

3. At the same time, drain the water from the jam jars, and set aside so that they are just warm when the soya milk has cooled.

4. Put half a teaspoonful of yogurt into each jar. Add a small amount of the tepid soya milk and mix to distribute the yogurt.

Then pour in the rest of the soya milk, filling the jars to the brim. Put on the lids and place the jars in a warm place for 6–8 hours, until the yogurt has set.

5. Let them cool, then put them into the fridge, where the yogurt will become even thicker. Save some of this batch to make the next batch.

> 0.4g carbs and 3.7g protein per 100ml (3½fl oz)

CEREALS

CRUNCHY GRANOLA

Phases 2/3 (V)
Preparation: 10 minutes

Serve this with hot or cold unsweetened soya milk, bought or home-made (see p. 145) or soya yogurt (see p. 147), or moisten with water and top with a little cream.

MAKES 6 SERVINGS
85g (3oz) flax seeds (linseeds)
85g (3oz) flax seeds (linseeds), ground
55g (2oz) desiccated coconut
55g (2oz) pumpkin seeds
55g (2oz) chopped or flaked almonds
½ teaspoon ground cinnamon (optional)

1. Mix all the ingredients together and keep in a sealed jar or container in the fridge.

> 4.7g carbs and 6g protein per serving
> (add extra carbs for the soya milk, yogurt or cream)

HIGH BRAN HOT CEREAL

Phases 1/2/3 Ⓥ
Preparation: 2–3 minutes

Wheat bran weighs very light, so the quantity may sound small but it gives a good bowlful. It's a comforting mixture – and also very helpful for constipation. You can flavour the basic mixture to your taste – some people like it salty, others prefer it slightly sweet. A dollop of soya yogurt (see p. 147) or soya cream are also good on it.

> **SERVES 1**
> 15g (½oz) wheat bran
> 2 tablespoons flax seeds (linseeds), finely ground
> 150–200ml (5–7fl oz) boiling water
> salt, stevia or low-carb sweetener, butter, ground cinnamon (to taste)

1. Put the wheat bran and ground flax seed into a bowl and add the boiling water. Stir, then let it stand for 2–3 minutes to let the cereal absorb the water.

2. Add the flavourings or toppings of your choice: a little salt, and a pat of butter, for instance, or a sprinkling of stevia or low-carb sweetener and a scattering of cinnamon.

> 3.1g carbs and 3.2g protein

SARA'S HOT CEREAL

Phases 2/3 Ⓥ
Preparation: 2–3 minutes / Cooking: 5 minutes

You can reduce the carb content of this hot cereal by leaving out the oats, which are pleasant but not essential.

MAKES 6 SERVINGS

55g (2oz) rolled oats (not 'instant' oats)

55g (2oz) finely ground almonds (bought ground, or powdered in an electric coffee grinder)

55g (2oz) chopped walnuts or hazelnuts

55g (2oz) wheatgerm (preferably not 'stabilised')

55g (2oz) soya protein isolate powder

6 tablespoons wheat bran

To serve:

150ml (5fl oz) boiling water

2 tablespoons freshly ground flax seeds (linseeds)

ground cinnamon, ground ginger, butter, cream and stevia or low-carb sweetener to taste

1. Spread the oats out on a grill pan and place under a hot grill for a few minutes until they smell toasted and turn a light golden-brown. Leave to cool.

2. Add the ground almonds, chopped nuts, wheatgerm, protein powder and wheat bran, and mix well. This is the basic mix: store in a sealed container in the fridge until required.

3. To use, put 3 rounded tablespoons of the mixture into a bowl and add the boiling water. Leave to soak for 1–2 minutes while you grind the flax seeds. Then stir them in, along with any of the other flavourings you choose: a sprinkling of ground cinnamon or ginger, a knob of butter, a spoonful of cream or soya cream, a little stevia or low-carb sweetener to taste.

> 10g carbs and 15.5g protein per serving
> (add extra carbs for the soya milk, yogurt or cream)

COOKED BREAKFAST DISHES

These are quick, simple and tasty – and most of them are things you could eat at any hour of the day.

SCRAMBLED EGGS ON A MUSHROOM

Phases 1/2/3
Preparation: 5 minutes / Cooking: 10 minutes

Scrambled eggs are luscious piled on a buttery, juicy mushroom. They are also excellent served on toasted Low-Carb Bread (see p. 294).

SERVES 1

2 eggs
1 tablespoon double cream
salt and freshly ground black pepper
2 knobs of butter and ½ tablespoon olive oil
1 large flat open mushroom, washed and blotted dry

1. Whisk the eggs with the cream and some salt and pepper and set aside.

2. Heat a knob of butter in a frying pan with the olive oil. Fry the mushroom, first on the black side, for a couple of minutes, then on the other side. Remove from the pan, put onto a plate and keep warm.

3. Wipe out the pan with a piece of kitchen paper, then put in another knob of butter and melt over a gentle heat.

4. Pour in the eggs. As they start to set around the edges, stir with a wooden spoon to make a creamy mixture. Once all the egg is set but still creamy, spoon it on top of the mushroom, and serve.

3.4g carbs and 16g protein

Vegan variation:

Make as above, substituting Scrambled Tofu (see below) for the scrambled eggs.

SCRAMBLED TOFU

Phases 1/2/3 Ⓥ

Preparation: 2–3 minutes / Cooking: 5 minutes

This is good served on a big mushroom (see previous recipe) or on Low-Carb Toast (see p. 294).

SERVES 1
1 tablespoon olive oil
28g (1oz) butter (or 2 more tablespoons of olive oil for vegan version)
½ packet or 125–140g (4½–5oz) firm tofu, drained and crumbled
½ teaspoon turmeric powder
2 tablespoons double cream or soya cream
salt and freshly ground black pepper
a little unsweetened soya milk (optional)

1. Heat the olive oil and butter, or just olive oil if making a vegan version, in a saucepan over a moderate heat.

2. Add the tofu, turmeric, cream and some salt and pepper to taste. Stir over a gentle heat until the tofu is hot and looks like scrambled egg.

3. If you like a runnier scramble, add a little unsweetened soya milk until you get the right consistency.

> 1.7g carbs and 21g protein

OMELETTE

Phases 1/2/3

Preparation: 2 minutes / Cooking: 2–3 minutes

An omelette is so quick and easy to make – and something you can enjoy at almost any time of the day. Here's the basic recipe, with some variations. Remember to get the filling ready before you start making the omelette, because it's done in a flash and best eaten at once.

SERVES 1

3 eggs
salt and freshly ground black pepper
20g (¾oz) butter, diced

1. Beat the eggs with a fork to break them up and combine. Season with salt and pepper, and stir in half the diced butter.

2. Heat the remaining butter in a medium frying pan over a high heat. When it foams, pour the egg mixture into the centre of the pan. Tip the pan so that the egg spreads all over the base. Then use a spatula to draw the set egg from the sides to the centre, and let the uncooked egg run from the centre towards the edges. Continue until the whole omelette is set.

3. Loosen the edges, fold the omelette over and turn it out.

> 1.2g carbs and 19g protein

Variations:

Cheese Omelette

Make as above, sprinkling 28g (1oz) grated Gruyère (or other cheese) on top of the omelette as soon as it has set. Fold over and serve. (Gruyère adds 0.1g carbs and 8.5g protein – for other types, see Carb and Protein Counter on pp. 312–8.)

Herb Omelette

Add chopped fresh herbs to the egg mixture before cooking: a tablespoonful each of chopped parsley, chopped chives and chopped tarragon – or whatever you fancy.

Watercress Omelette

Put several sprigs of fresh watercress on top of the omelette after it has set, fold it over and serve. The watercress gives a nice crunchy contrast to the buttery omelette.

Mushroom Omelette

Fry 28–55g (1–2oz) mushrooms and a crushed garlic clove in a little butter and olive oil in the frying pan for about 5 minutes, until the mushrooms are tender. Remove them from the pan, make the omelette as described, put the mushrooms on top, and fold over. (Adds about 1.5g carbs and negligible extra protein.)

Asparagus Omelette

Make the omelette as described, then top with 3–4 hot, cooked asparagus spears, fold over and serve. (Adds about 1.5g carbs and negligible extra protein.)

> 13–19g protein and 1–1.5g carbs, depending on number of eggs used (allow extra carbs for the fillings but none of the suggestions here add more than 2g carbs)

OVEN-BAKED MUSHROOM FRITTATA

Phases 1/2/3
Preparation: 10 minutes / Cooking: 15 minutes

This is a wonderful low-carb breakfast or snack and is as good cold as it is hot, so it makes a useful portable meal.

MAKES 12 PIECES
15g (½oz) butter
1 tablespoon olive oil
500g (1lb 2oz) mushrooms, washed and sliced
2 garlic cloves, peeled and chopped or crushed
salt and freshly ground black pepper
6 eggs, whisked
28g (1oz) Gruyère cheese, finely grated

1. Preheat the oven to 200°C (400°F) Gas Mark 6. Line a shallow 23 × 33cm (9 × 13in) tin with a strip of non-stick baking paper to cover the base and sides.

2. Heat the butter and oil in a large saucepan. Put in the mushrooms and garlic and fry over the heat for 10–15 minutes until they are tender and any liquid that they produce has boiled away. Season with salt and pepper.

3. Spread the mushrooms evenly over the base of the tin, on top of the paper.

4. Season the beaten eggs, then pour them over the mushrooms. Sprinkle the grated cheese over the top.

5. Bake for about 15 minutes, or until set, lightly browned and puffy. Cut into 12 pieces and eat hot or cold.

1g carbs and 5g protein per slice

OVEN-BAKED VEGAN MUSHROOM FRITTATA

Phases 1/2/3
Preparation: 10 minutes / Cooking: 15 minutes

You can also make a very good vegan version of the Oven-baked Mushroom Frittata ...

MAKES 8 PIECES
2 tablespoons olive oil
500g (1lb 2oz) mushrooms, washed and sliced
2 garlic cloves, peeled and chopped or crushed
salt and freshly ground black pepper
2 × 250g firm tofu, drained and broken into chunks
½ teaspoon turmeric
4 tablespoons plain unsweetened soya milk (bought or home-made, see p. 145)

1. Preheat the oven to 200°C (400°F) Gas Mark 6. Line a shallow 23 × 33cm (9 × 13in) tin with a strip of non-stick baking paper to cover the base and sides.

2. Heat the oil in a large saucepan. Put in the mushrooms and garlic and fry over the heat for 10–15 minutes until they are tender and any liquid that they produce has boiled away. Season with salt and pepper.

3. Spread the mushrooms evenly over the base of the tin, on top of the paper.

4. Whiz the tofu in a food processor with the turmeric, soya milk and some salt and pepper, until smooth and creamy. Pour over the mushrooms, allowing the mixture to spread to the edges.

5. Bake for 30 minutes, until firm. Cut into 8 slices.

1.6g carbs and 7.2g protein per slice

FLAKY SMOKED TOFU

Phases 1/2/3 Ⓥ
Preparation: 5 minutes / Cooking: 5 minutes

This is a very simple recipe, particularly enjoyed by vegetarians or vegans who fancy the smoky flavour and tender, flaky consistency of kippers or haddock. Try it with some fried mushrooms and grilled tomato.

SERVES 1
1 × 225g (8oz) packet smoked tofu, drained
15g (½oz) butter or 1 tablespoon olive oil
salt and freshly ground black pepper

To serve:
chopped parsley (optional)
lemon wedge

1. Cut the tofu into very thin flakes. The slicing edge of a grater is excellent for this, or you could use a knife, but make them as fine and flaky as you can.

2. Heat the butter or oil in a small saucepan, add the tofu and toss over the heat for a few minutes until heated through and shiny with the butter or oil.

3. Season with salt and plenty of pepper. Serve sprinkled with chopped parsley, if using, and a lemon wedge.

2.2g carbs and 35g protein

PANCAKES

Phases 1/2/3

Preparation: 10 minutes / Cooking: 10 minutes

Pancakes for breakfast – on a diet? Yes, you really can treat yourself to these.

> **MAKES 4–6 PANCAKES**
>
> 100g (3½oz) low- or medium-fat cream cheese
> 2 eggs
> 1 tablespoon soya protein isolate powder
> ½ teaspoon baking powder
> a pinch of salt
> 1 teaspoon vanilla or almond extract (optional)
> olive oil
>
> **To serve:**
> a sprinkling of stevia or sugar, or no-carb maple syrup, or a teaspoonful
> of honey dissolved in a little hot water, or some berries sweetened
> with a little stevia

1. Blend the cream cheese and eggs together in a bowl until smooth. Sprinkle the soya powder, baking powder and salt over the top and whisk until smooth. Stir in the vanilla or almond extract if using.

2. Smear some olive oil over a frying pan using some kitchen paper, then heat the frying pan. When it's sizzling hot, pour in enough of the batter to coat the base of the frying pan lightly, tipping the pan so that the mixture flows all over it. Cook for a few seconds, until the underneath is lightly browned and the top is set.

3. Flip the pancake over, using a palette knife or a spatula, and cook for a few seconds longer. Remove from the pan and repeat until all the batter is used.

> 8g carbs and 32g protein for the whole quantity

SPINACH 'BREAD'

Phases 1/2/3
Preparation: 15 minutes / Cooking 10–15 minutes

Although the idea of green 'bread' may seem weird at first, I assure you it's wonderful. You can spread the cooled 'bread' with cream cheese or mayonnaise and fillings of your choice, topping it with another piece for wonderful green sandwiches. Or try spreading it with tomato sauce, grated cheese and any toppings you like, then putting it under the grill for green 'pizza'. It's also great as a base for toasted cheese.

I've adapted this from a Suzanne Somers recipe. You can use a Swiss roll tin measuring either 33 × 23cm (13 × 9in) or 35 × 25cm (14 × 10in) for this; the larger tin gives a slightly thinner 'bread', takes a few minutes less time to bake, and cuts into slightly larger pieces.

280g (10oz) frozen chopped spinach, defrosted
4 eggs, beaten
1 garlic clove, peeled and crushed
salt and freshly ground black pepper

1. Preheat the oven to 180°C (350°F) Gas Mark 4. Line your chosen Swiss roll tin with a piece of non-stick paper.

2. Squeeze as much liquid out of the defrosted spinach as you can. (Try squashing it into a fine-mesh sieve with the back of a spoon.) Then mix it in a bowl with the eggs, garlic and some salt and pepper.

3. Pour the mixture into the tin, smoothing it into the corners. Bake for 10–15 minutes, until firm and springy.

4. Leave to cool in the tin, then cut into pieces.

> 5.8g carbs and 36g protein for the whole quantity
> 1g carb and 6g protein per slice (for 6 slices)

Variation:
If you don't like garlic, replace the clove with a pinch of nutmeg.

10

Quick Lunches and Snacks

Lunch, like breakfast, is a versatile meal and can be anything you want it to be – soup, salad, low-carb sandwiches – just make sure you get it. In fact, it can't be said too often: don't skip any meals, and make sure you include enough protein – at least 20g at every meal if you're a woman, 25g if you're a man.

Here are some ideas for quick lunches:

- A bowl of soup and some Low-Carb Bread (see p. 294), or Almond Crackers (see p. 296), with some vegan or dairy cheese.

- Any of the salads in this section (see pp. 171–82).

- A Low-Carb Vegeburger (see p. 209) or slice of Nut Roast (see p. 249) or any left-over savoury from the night before, with some green salad leaves.

- Crunchy Tofu Sticks (see p. 206), with Mayonnaise (see p. 187) or Avocado Dip (see p. 200).

- A 'fast food' lunch, just for fun: Turnip Chips (see p. 264) with a Low-Carb Vegeburger (see p. 209) and some Easy Tomato Ketchup (see p. 189).

Some of the suggestions above will travel well – you just need a good range of airtight containers – but here are some more ideas specifically for packed lunches:

- Devilled Eggs (see p. 193), on their own or with some salad.

- Cold Omelette (see p. 153).

- Sandwiches made with Spinach 'Bread' (see p. 159) and cream cheese or a chopped hard-boiled egg mixed with mayonnaise, or avocado and tomato, or cheese – any filling you might normally use between slices of bread. You could also use high-protein, Low-Carb Bread (see p. 294) to make sandwiches in the same way.

- Salad wraps – roll large, flexible lettuce leaves around any of the following: cream cheese, chopped avocado, egg salad or Tofu 'Egg' Mayonnaise (see p. 183), peanut butter and cream cheese (or soya yogurt or Vegan Cream Cheese, see p. 199); peanut butter with chopped celery and a little grated carrot; or Marinated Tofu (see p. 219).

- Sesame and Tofu Hummus (see p. 198) or Tofu Mayonnaise (see p. 188) or any other low-carb, protein-rich dip, with crudités, e.g. celery sticks, strips of green pepper, mangetouts, radishes, chicory leaves, pieces of fresh fennel, Little Gem lettuce hearts.

- A bag of salad leaves and some cubes of cheese – up to 100g (3½oz), using your whole day's 'ration' of cheese.

- A tub of plain unsweetened soya yogurt, bought or home-made (see p. 147), and 28g (1oz) almonds.

- A protein shake (just take the powder in a screw-top plastic cup and shake it with water when required) and a vegetable salad. There's no need to think about the protein content of the salad if you have the shake.

- A piece of Mushroom Quiche (see p. 253), with salad.

- Left-overs from your previous evening's meal can be eaten cold or reheated in a microwave if available. Or you could make up a batch of a favourite dish especially for lunches – such as Low-Carb Pizza (see p. 255) – divide it into portions and freeze it in suitable containers.

- Bought vegeburgers or vegetarian sausages, which you can microwave or grill and eat with a salad that you've packed.

SOUPS

A cup or bowl of soup is great for lunch in cold weather. Some of the soups that follow, such as Tomato Cheddar Soup or Celery and Blue Cheese Soup, contain enough protein to be the main source for the meal.

Other soups, such as Vegetable Soup, can have protein added in the form of grated cheese. Or you can serve them with a slice of protein-rich Low-Carb Bread (see p. 294) or a Spinach 'Bread' sandwich (see p. 159), a slice of Mushroom Quiche (see p. 253), or a protein-rich dip, salad or pudding.

TOMATO CHEDDAR SOUP

Phases 1/2/3

Preparation: 5 minutes / Cooking: 25 minutes

A vegetarian low-carber gave me this soup recipe, which I've adapted slightly. It makes a creamy, protein-rich soup, and you can freeze it too.

SERVES 4

1 × 400g (14oz) can tomatoes
2 celery stalks, roughly chopped
1 small onion, peeled and roughly chopped
1 garlic clove, peeled and crushed
700ml (1¼ pints) water
1 teaspoon dried basil
250ml (9fl oz) unsweetened soya cream
225g (8oz) Cheddar cheese, grated
salt and freshly ground black pepper

1. Put the tomatoes in a food processor with the celery, onion and garlic, and whiz until smooth.

2. Pour into a large saucepan and add the water and basil. Bring to the boil and simmer, uncovered, for 20 minutes.

3. Stir in the soya cream and grated cheese, and season with salt and pepper. Gently bring to the boil, stirring, as the cheese melts. Serve at once.

6.2g carbs and 16.3g protein per serving

CREAMY CAULIFLOWER SOUP

Phases 1/2/3 Ⓥ

Preparation: 10 minutes / Cooking: 15 minutes

Smooth and creamy, this is a low-carb replacement for that wonderful comfort food, potato soup.

SERVES 6

2 tablespoons olive oil

2 celery sticks, finely chopped

1 onion, peeled and finely chopped

1 large cauliflower, cut into small pieces

1.3 litres (2¼ pints) water

2 bay leaves

100ml (3½fl oz) unsweetened soya cream or double cream

salt and freshly ground black pepper

grated nutmeg

1. Heat the oil in a saucepan, add the celery and onion, stir and cover. Cook gently for 10–15 minutes, until tender.

2. Meanwhile, cook the cauliflower in the water with the bay leaves for about 10 minutes, or until tender. Discard the bay leaves.

3. Liquidise the cauliflower, and its cooking water, with the onion and celery mixture, to make a smooth soup. Stir in the cream and season with salt, pepper and grated nutmeg.

7g carbs and 3.7g protein per serving

CELERY AND BLUE CHEESE SOUP

Phases 1/2/3
Preparation: 10 minutes / Cooking: 30 minutes

This creamy soup, with the tang of blue cheese, contains a useful amount of protein.

SERVES 4
500g (1lb 2oz) celery, roughly chopped
1 small onion, peeled and roughly chopped
850ml (1½ pints) water
150g (5½oz) blue cheese, crumbled
salt and freshly ground black pepper

To serve:
4 tablespoons double cream
chopped chives

1. Put the celery and onion in a food processor with the water and whiz until smooth.

2. Pour into a large saucepan, bring to the boil, cover and simmer for about 30 minutes, until the celery is very tender.

3. Add the crumbled cheese, stirring gently over the heat until smooth and creamy. Season with salt and pepper and reheat gently.

4. Serve each portion with a swirl of cream and some chopped chives on top.

> 4.1g carbs and 9.3g protein per serving

QUICK SPINACH SOUP

Phases 1/2/3 Ⓥ
Preparation: 10 minutes / Cooking: 10 minutes

Keep a bag of frozen spinach in the freezer and you can make this soup in an instant.

SERVES 2
1 onion, about 55g (2oz), peeled and chopped
1 tablespoon olive oil
150g (5½oz) frozen chopped spinach
1 garlic clove, peeled and crushed
300ml (½ pint) soya milk, bought or home-made (see p. 145)
2 tablespoons double cream or soya cream
salt and freshly ground black pepper
grated nutmeg

1. Fry the onion in the olive oil in a large saucepan, covered, for about 7 minutes, or until tender.

2. Add the spinach and garlic, stir over the heat for 1–2 minutes, then add the soya milk, cream and salt, pepper and nutmeg to taste. Reheat, but don't boil, then serve.

3. If you want the soup to be smoother, give it a whiz in a food processor or with a stick blender before serving.

> 4.4g carbs and 9g protein per serving

CREAMY MUSHROOM SOUP

Phases 1/2/3 **Ⓥ**
Preparation: 15 minutes / Cooking: 30 minutes

This is a lovely, creamy soup, high in protein, which can make a complete meal. It's quick to make but does not freeze well.

SERVES 2
1 small onion, peeled and finely chopped
1 tablespoon olive oil
150g (5½oz) mushrooms, washed and sliced
250g (9oz) firm tofu, drained
1 garlic clove, peeled
1 teaspoon vegetable bouillon or stock powder
225ml (8fl oz) water
salt and freshly ground black pepper
soy sauce (to taste)

1. Fry the onion in the olive oil in a large saucepan for about 5 minutes, or until beginning to soften. Add the mushrooms and cook for a further 4–5 minutes, until the mushrooms are cooked.

2. Meanwhile, put the tofu, garlic, vegetable bouillon or stock powder and water into a food processor or blender and whiz thoroughly until very smooth.

3. Add the tofu mixture to the mushrooms in the pan and heat gently. Add a little more water if necessary to get the consistency you want, then season with salt, pepper and a dash of soy sauce, and serve.

5.5g carbs and 27.5g protein

QUICK VEGETABLE SOUP

Phases 1/2/3 Ⓥ

Preparation: 15 minutes / Cooking: 30 minutes

This is a lovely, warming, filling soup, which can make a very satisfying lunch if you add grated cheese (or crisp-fried tofu or tempeh for vegans) and some protein-rich Low-Carb Bread (see p. 294). Making a big batch of this at the weekend can be a lifesaver when you need to make quick meals during the week.

SERVES 4

1 small onion, peeled and chopped
1 tablespoon olive oil
1 garlic clove, peeled and crushed
1 turnip, peeled and cut into 1cm (½in) dice
½ Chinese cabbage (Chinese leaves), sliced
1 × 400g (14oz) can tomatoes
600ml (1 pint) water
1 teaspoon vegetable bouillon powder
1 × 425g (15oz) can fine green beans, drained
1 × 400g (14oz) can celery hearts, drained and cut into large chunks
salt and freshly ground black pepper
chopped parsley or torn basil leaves (optional)

1. Fry the onion in the olive oil in a large saucepan, covered, for about 7 minutes, or until tender.

2. Add the garlic, turnip and cabbage, and stir over the heat for 1–2 minutes. Then add the tomatoes, water and bouillon powder.

3. Bring to the boil and simmer for about 10 minutes, or until the vegetables are tender.

4. Roughly purée using a stick blender, or purée a cupful or so of the mixture in a food processor and return to the pan – the aim is to thicken the soup a bit while still keeping plenty of texture.

5. Add the green beans and celery hearts and bring back to the boil. Season with salt and pepper – you won't need much salt, because the canned vegetables will add some. Serve with some chopped parsley or torn basil on top, if available.

6. This is even better the next day – and can also be livened up with some chilli powder for a slightly different flavour.

9.5g carbs and 4g protein per serving

SALADS

A salad is a convenient meal to have at lunchtime – or at any time of the day. It's quick and easy to put together, delicious, crunchy and healthy, and can be as nutritious and filling as a cooked dish. Most vegetables can be eaten freely on the Vegetarian Low-Carb Diet, certainly once you're past the first fortnight, so there's lots of scope for using different ingredients.

A home-made Vinaigrette (see p. 185) can be counted as 0g carbs. If you use bought vinaigrette, make sure you check the carbs on the label – but you should be able to get a very, very low one. Again, for bought mayonnaise, you need to check the label. Most good-quality brands contain almost no carbs. My favourite one is Hellmann's. I've also given a recipe for home-made Mayonnaise (see p. 187) for those who prefer to make their own. This does have a slight carb content but it's so low that it barely makes any difference.

BIG-LEAF SALAD WITH EVERYTHING IN IT

Phases 2/3
Preparation: 10 minutes

Use whatever mixture of salad leaves you like for this – lettuce, baby spinach, rocket, watercress – and top with your favourite low-carb ingredients. The following is just a suggestion.

SERVES 1
85g (3oz) mixed salad leaves
vinaigrette, bought or home-made (see p. 185, optional)
55–85g (2–3oz) Cheddar cheese, grated
15g (½oz) pumpkin seeds or walnuts
½ red pepper, sliced
8 cherry tomatoes, halved
chopped chives or some torn leaves of basil

1. Line a large plate with the lettuce leaves and drizzle with a little vinaigrette if you like.

2. Top with the grated cheese, pumpkin seeds or walnuts, red pepper, cherry tomatoes and the fresh herbs. Drizzle with a little more vinaigrette if you wish, and serve at once.

> 10.2g carbs and 27.5g protein

Vegan variation:
Use vegan Cheddar cheese – check the carbs.

GREEK SALAD

Phases 2/3
Preparation: 10 minutes

SERVES 1
25g (1oz) lettuce, shredded
vinaigrette, bought or home-made (see p. 185, optional)
5cm (2in) cucumber, diced
1 medium tomato, diced
½ green pepper, de-seeded and sliced
15g (½oz) onion, thinly sliced
5–6 Kalamata olives
55g (2oz) Feta cheese, diced

1. Line a large plate with the lettuce leaves and drizzle with a little vinaigrette if you like.

2. Mix together all the remaining ingredients – the cucumber, tomato, green pepper, onion, olives and Feta, and toss in a little vinaigrette.

3. Pile the mixture on top of the lettuce, and serve at once.

> 10g carbs and 10.4g protein

Vegan variation:
Use vegan Feta or small pieces of vegan cream cheese – check the carbs.

SALADE NIÇOISE

Phases 2/3
Preparation: 10 minutes

I love to serve this as a warm salad, by mixing everything with the beans as soon as they're done, but it's equally good served cold, the traditional way – and you can use canned French beans in an emergency.

SERVES 1
115g (4oz) slim French beans, very lightly trimmed, or just left as they
  are
2 hard-boiled eggs, sliced
1 tomato, sliced
5–6 Kalamata olives
28g (1oz) onion, peeled and finely sliced
vinaigrette, bought or home-made (see p. 185, optional)

1. Cook the French beans in a little fast-boiling water for about 5 minutes, or until they are just tender; drain.

2. Mix the beans with all the other ingredients – the hard-boiled eggs, tomato, olives and onion, and add vinaigrette if you wish. Toss lightly, and serve.

> 16g carbs and 10.6g protein

Vegan variation:
Use marinated tofu – home-made (see p. 219) or bought (check the carbs) instead of the hard-boiled eggs.

CAESAR SALAD

Phases 1/2/3
Preparation: 10 minutes

A low-carb vegetarian – or vegan – Caesar salad needs a bit of innovation, but can be great. Give the mayonnaise a good kick with plenty of Tabasco to replace the tang of the traditional anchovies, and, instead of the croûtons, use a few crunchy toasted flaked almonds or macadamia nuts. It's particularly good with freshly toasted almonds tossed in at the last minute, still hot from the grill. Use a Parmesan-style Parmesan to be sure this is vegetarian.

SERVES 1
½ Romaine lettuce (about 85g/3oz)
1 heaped tablespoon mayonnaise, bought or home-made (see p. 187)
a few drops of Tabasco
55g (2oz) Parmesan cheese, cut into thin flakes
15g (½oz) flaked almonds, toasted, or macadamia nuts

1. Line a serving bowl with the lettuce leaves, arranging them around the edge, with a space in the middle for the mayonnaise.

2. Mix the mayonnaise with the Tabasco and half the Parmesan. Spoon into the centre of the salad and scatter with the rest of the cheese and the flaked almonds or macadamia nuts.

> 4.6g carbs and 25g protein

Vegan variation:
Use grated vegan 'Parmesan' which you can buy in a little tub. You'll only need half the quantity, as it's very powdery, so increase the nuts instead, and check the carbs.

CHICORY AND WATERCRESS SALAD WITH BLUE CHEESE DRESSING

Phases 1/2/3
Preparation: 10 minutes

You can really use whatever salad leaves you fancy to provide a base for this tangy creamy dressing. I particularly like it over crisp, crunchy chicory and 'hot' watercress – and the fact that they have just about the lowest carbs of any vegetable adds to the appeal for me.

SERVES 1
1 head of chicory, about 100g (3½oz), separated into leaves
55g (2oz) watercress
100g (3½oz) blue cheese, crumbled
2 tablespoons soya milk, water or plain yogurt
15g (½oz) walnuts, toasted

1. Cover a plate with the chicory and watercress.

2. Mix the crumbled blue cheese with the soya milk, water or yogurt, to make a creamy dressing.

3. Spoon the dressing over the salad, and sprinkle with the nuts.

> 4.7g carbs and 25.6g protein

Vegan variation:
Use a vegan blue cheese, finely grated, with soya yogurt or soya cream, to mix. Check the carbs.

ROASTED VEGETABLE SALAD

Phases 2/3
Preparation: 10 minutes

This is a very easy main meal salad if you make a double batch of Roasted Vegetables and save half.

> **SERVES 1**
> 55g (2oz) rocket
> ½ quantity Roasted Vegetables (see p. 265)
> a little red wine vinegar
> salt and freshly ground black pepper
> 55g (2oz) shaved Parmesan-style cheese
> a sprig of basil, torn

1. Cover a plate with the rocket.

2. Mix the roasted vegetables with a few drops of red wine vinegar and some salt and pepper to taste. (Or you could use a little vinaigrette, but I find the oil from the vegetables blends well with the vinegar to make its own dressing.)

3. Spoon the vegetables on top of the rocket and top with the Parmesan and basil. Serve at once.

> 17g carbs and 26g protein

Vegan variation:
Use a vegan cheese, or some marinated tofu, instead of the Parmesan-style cheese. Count the carbs.

MEXICAN SALAD

Phases 2/3

Preparation: 10 minutes

This is one where you can more or less throw everything in (as long as you count the carbs!) and it makes a big, main meal salad. You can spice up the vegemince with some chilli powder if you wish.

SERVES 1

55g (2oz) Iceberg lettuce, shredded
½ red pepper, sliced
1 tomato, sliced
28g (1oz) onion, peeled and thinly sliced
100g (3½oz) vegetarian mince
a small piece of chilli, sliced
1 tablespoon olive oil
½ avocado, peeled and chopped
2 tablespoons soured cream
salt and freshly ground black pepper

1. Cover a plate with the shredded lettuce. Arrange the red pepper, tomato and onion slices over the top.

2. Fry the mince and chilli in the olive oil, stirring for a few minutes until heated through.

3. Spoon the chilli mince on top of the salad, then top with the chopped avocado and the soured cream – or offer these separately. Serve at once.

18g carbs and 22g protein

Vegan variation:

Use vegan cream, soured with a few drops of wine vinegar, instead of soured cream, or a dollop or two of vegan yogurt.

ROCKET AND PARMESAN SALAD

Phases 1/2/3
Preparation: 10 minutes

This is a restaurant favourite that's become a classic.

SERVES 1
85g (3oz) rocket
1–2 tablespoons vinaigrette, bought or home-made (see p. 185)
55g (2oz) Parmesan-style cheese, shaved

1. Put the rocket into a bowl with the vinaigrette and toss gently, until all the leaves are lightly coated.

2. Add the Parmesan shavings, toss again, and serve heaped up on a plate.

Vegan variation:
Use thinly sliced vegan Cheddar cheese instead of the Parmesan-style cheese.

> 3.6g carbs and 22.3g protein

SOFT GOAT'S CHEESE SALAD WITH PECAN NUTS

Phases 1/2/3
Preparation: 10 minutes / Cooking: 3–4 minutes

When you buy the goat's cheese, be sure to check the carbs on the label, as they do vary, and buy the very lowest you can find. I used a 0g carbs one for this recipe. If you can't find a low one, either add the carbs to the count given, or use another cheese such as a semi-soft goat's cheese or Brie. The pecan nuts taste extra-good if you toast them just before serving the salad, and add them when they're hot and sizzling. But this isn't essential – it's delicious anyway.

SERVES 1
85g (3oz) lettuce (preferably red oakleaf, endive or chicory)
a few chopped fresh herbs (e.g. chervil and chives), optional
vinaigrette, bought or home-made (see p. 185)
85g (3oz) soft goat's cheese, broken into pieces
28g (1oz) pecan nuts, roughly chopped

1. Cover a plate with the lettuce or other leaves, scatter with herbs if using, drizzle with a little vinaigrette, and dot the goat's cheese over the top.

2. Put the pecan nuts onto a grill pan and toast under a hot grill for 1–2 minutes until they smell delicious and are lightly browned. Watch them carefully, as they burn quickly.

3. Remove the pecans from the heat as soon as they're ready and toss over the top of the salad. Serve at once.

> 2.2g carbs and 24g protein

HOT GOAT'S CHEESE SALAD

Phases 1/2/3
Preparation: 10 minutes / Cooking: 5–10 minutes

Usually in this French bistro salad, the goat's cheese is melted on top of slices of baguette, and piled on top of the salad. However you can make a great low-carb version by simply melting the goat's cheese under the grill, then scooping the hot, browned, sizzling cheese on top of the salad leaves. When you buy the goat's cheese, be sure to check the carbs on the label, as they do vary, and buy the very lowest you can find. I used a 0g carbs one for this recipe. If you can't find a low one, add the carbs to the count given.

SERVES 1
100g (3½oz) round of chevre blanc goat's cheese
85g (3oz) lettuce, e.g. red oakleaf or any other type, or watercress
a few chopped fresh herbs (e.g. chervil and chives), optional
vinaigrette, bought or home-made (see p. 185)
5–6 Kalamata olives

1. If you've got the large, flat goat's cheese, slice it horizontally, to make two thin, round pieces. If you've got the smaller, taller little goat's cheeses, you may be able to get three or four slices out of each.

2. Line the grill pan with some non-stick tin foil, lay the slices of goat's cheese on the foil and put them under a hot grill.

3. Meanwhile toss the lettuce, or whichever leaves you're using, and the herbs if available, in vinaigrette, and put onto a large plate. Dot with the olives.

4. When the goat's cheese is golden brown, melted and sizzling, with crisp bits round the edges, use a spatula to scrape it off the foil and put on top of the salad. Eat at once.

> 2.2g carbs and 24g protein

AVOCADO, COTTAGE CHEESE AND SPINACH SALAD

Phases 1/2/3

Preparation: 10 minutes

Cottage cheese doesn't feature much in the low-carb diet, because it's a bit carby compared to many other cheeses. However, it has its own charm, so it's nice to include it sometimes, and I particularly like it in this salad, where it contrasts well with the creamy, buttery avocado.

SERVES 1

55g (2oz) rocket or watercress
vinaigrette, bought or home-made (see p. 185)
15g (½oz) walnuts
½ avocado, peeled and chopped
salt and freshly ground black pepper
55g (2oz) cottage cheese

1. Cover a plate with the rocket or watercress and drizzle with a little vinaigrette; scatter with the walnuts.

2. Put the avocado on top of the leaves, season with salt and pepper, then spoon the cottage cheese into the cavity. Serve at once.

Vegan variation:

Use vegan cream cheese instead of cottage cheese.

6g carbs and 13g protein

MIMOSA SALAD

Phases 1/2/3
Preparation: 10 minutes / Cooking: 10 minutes

This is a particularly attractive version of egg salad, with the delicate flavour of tarragon (or chives if you can't get tarragon).

SERVES 1
2 eggs
1 tablespoon mayonnaise, bought or home-made (see p. 187)
1 tablespoon chopped fresh tarragon or chives
heart of 1 small round lettuce, plus 3–4 outer leaves
salt and freshly ground black pepper

1. Boil the eggs for 10 minutes, until hard-boiled. Drain and put under cold running water to cool quickly, then peel off the shells.

2. Remove one egg yolk and set aside. Finely chop or grate the rest of the eggs and mix with the mayonnaise and tarragon or chives.

3. Line a bowl with the lettuce leaves. Spoon the egg mixture into the centre. Grate or mash the remaining egg yolk and sprinkle over the top.

> 2g carbs and 14g protein

TOFU 'EGG' MAYONNAISE

Phases 1/2/3 **Ⓥ**

Preparation: 10 minutes (plus 1 hour optional standing time)

This tastes remarkably like normal Egg Mayonnaise. Use the vegan version of mayonnaise (see p. 188) for a lovely vegan lunch or low-carb starter for a dinner party.

SERVES 1

125g (4½oz) firm tofu
¼ teaspoon ground turmeric
1 tablespoon mayonnaise, bought or home-made (see p. 187)
¼ teaspoon Dijon mustard
1 tablespoon chopped celery
salt and freshly ground black pepper

To serve:
2–3 lettuce leaves
1 tablespoon chopped chives

1. Drain and mash the tofu, then mix with the turmeric, mayonnaise, mustard, chopped celery and salt and pepper.

2. Leave to stand for an hour to allow the flavours to develop, or serve at once – make a base of the lettuce leaves, spoon the tofu 'egg' mayonnaise into the centre and top with the chives.

> 2g carbs and 20g protein

COLESLAW

Phases 1/2/3 **Ⓥ**
Preparation: 10 minutes

It's easy to make your own coleslaw and avoid the sugar or artificial sweetenings that may have been added to bought versions. This coleslaw keeps for several days in a covered container in the fridge, so it may be worth making up a larger quantity. A food processor with a grating attachment makes light work of the chopping, although if you use a tender cabbage, such as one of the light-green pointed varieties, they're quite easy to shred with a sharp knife. When you're past Phase 1 of the diet you could add a little grated carrot to this recipe – allow 1.9 carbs for 28g (1oz) carrot. Serve this with vegetarian sausages, eggs or tofu to make a complete meal.

SERVES 1

100g (3½oz) cabbage, core trimmed away
1 spring onion, chopped
1 celery stick, sliced
½ teaspoon Dijon mustard
1 tablespoon mayonnaise, bought or home-made (see p. 187)
salt and freshly ground black pepper
1 tablespoon unsweetened dairy yogurt or soya yogurt (optional)

1. Shred the cabbage finely. Mix the cabbage, spring onion, celery, mustard and mayonnaise in a bowl, then season with salt and pepper. If you like a creamier consistency, stir in the yogurt.

> 5.5g carbs and 3.3g protein

DRESSINGS AND SAUCES

Dressings and sauces, both hot and cold, can make many dishes tastier and more appetising. And some of them, such as Coconut Sauce, can even form the basis of a quick meal (see the Egg Curry recipe on p. 226).

VINAIGRETTE

Phases 1/2/3 Ⓥ

Making your own dressing is easy, and if you do it yourself you know what's in it and can keep it carb-free. Mix it up in a screw-top bottle or jar and keep it handy in the fridge.

> **MAKES 125ML (4FL OZ)**
> salt and freshly ground black pepper
> 1 teaspoon Dijon mustard (optional)
> 4 tablespoons red wine vinegar
> 8 tablespoons olive oil

1. Put a teaspoonful of salt, a good grinding of black pepper, and the Dijon mustard, if using, into a screw-top bottle or jar. Add the vinegar and shake to blend, then add the olive oil and shake again.

2. Keep in the fridge and use as required. The olive oil may thicken up a bit in the cold, but it will soon return to normal at room temperature. Shake it before using.

> trace carbs and trace protein

YOGURT DRESSING

Phases 1/2/3 **Ⓥ**
Preparation: 5 minutes

This is another recipe that's useful to make up and keep in the fridge, to save time during the week. I like to use soya yogurt, but it also works well, for non-vegans, with dairy yogurt and with soured cream – you'll need to check the carbs on the cartons if you use these.

> **MAKES 300ML (10FL OZ)**
> 300ml (10fl oz) soya yogurt, bought or home-made (see p. 147)
> 1 tablespoon olive oil
> 2 tablespoons chopped fresh herbs
> salt and freshly ground black pepper
> a few drops of red wine vinegar (optional)

1. Beat the soya yogurt to break up any lumps, then stir in the olive oil, until combined.

2. Stir in the chopped herbs and add salt, pepper, and vinegar if using, to taste.

> 7.2g carbs and 13.5g protein for the whole amount
> 0.4g carbs and 0.7g protein per tablespoonful

MAYONNAISE

Phases 1/2/3

Preparation: 2 minutes

Making your own mayonnaise means you can use the best-quality, healthiest oil and avoid sugar and other unwanted additives. Use a fresh, organic free-range egg from a source you trust. I make this with a stick blender straight in the jug in which I measure the oil, but you can also use a blender or food processor.

NOTE: It's best not to use raw eggs if you're pregnant or feeling at all unwell. Use the vegan variation instead – it's yummy.

MAKES 250ML (9FL OZ)

200ml (7fl oz) extra-virgin olive oil

1 large organic free-range egg

2 garlic cloves, peeled and crushed

1 teaspoon Dijon mustard

1 tablespoon red wine vinegar

½ teaspoon salt (or to taste)

freshly ground black pepper

1. Put the oil, egg, garlic, mustard, vinegar, salt and pepper into a blender or food processor and whiz for a few seconds until thick, pale and creamy. Or add all the ingredients to the oil in a deep measuring jug and whiz with a stick blender. Transfer to a lidded jar and keep in the fridge for up to a month.

> 2.6g carbs and 6.7g protein for whole quantity
> (0.16g carbs and 0.4g protein per tablespoonful)

Vegan variation:

Make exactly as described but use 4 tablespoons soya milk or soya cream instead of the egg.

> 3.0g carbs and 2.7g protein for whole quantity
> (0.2g carbs and 0.16g protein per tablespoonful)

TOFU MAYONNAISE

Phases 1/2/3 **V**
Preparation: 6 minutes

This is a rich source of protein – it can turn a plain, crisp salad into a main meal.

SERVES 2–4
250g (9oz) firm tofu, drained and broken into pieces
1 tablespoon Dijon mustard
2 tablespoons red wine vinegar
2 tablespoons olive oil
salt and freshly ground black pepper

1. Put the tofu into a food processor or blender with the mustard, vinegar, oil and some salt and pepper. Whiz until you get a thick, creamy consistency.

> 3g carbs and 40g protein for the whole quantity
> (0.15g carbs and 2g protein per tablespoonful)

EASY TOMATO KETCHUP

Phases 1/2/3 Ⓥ

Preparation: 2 minutes

This low-carb version tastes very much like the real thing.

MAKES 200ML (7FL OZ)

100ml (3½fl oz) tomato purée

100ml (3½fl oz) wine vinegar, red or white

1–2 teaspoons dried oregano

salt

stevia or low-carb sweetener (to taste)

1. Mix together the tomato purée and vinegar. Add the oregano, salt and a dash of stevia or sweetener to taste.

2. This will keep well in a sealed container in the fridge, because the vinegar is a natural preservative.

> 12.2g carbs and 4.1g protein for the whole amount
> (about 1g carbs and 0.4g protein per tablespoonful)

GRAVY

Phases 1/2/3
Preparation: 5 minutes / Cooking: 10 minutes

As well as being very low in carbs, this gravy is a great way of adding extra protein to a meal.

SERVES 2–3
2 tablespoons olive oil
55g (2oz) onion, peeled and finely chopped
28g (1oz) soya protein isolate powder
300ml (10fl oz) water
2 tablespoons soy sauce
1 teaspoon vegetable bouillon powder

1. Heat the oil in a saucepan, add the onion, cover and cook for about 7 minutes, or until tender and lightly browned.

2. Stir in the soya isolate powder, then add the water, stirring all the time. Add the soy sauce and bouillon powder, allow to simmer gently for 2–3 minutes, and serve.

> 5g carbs and 26g protein for the whole quantity
> (0.27g carbs and 1.3g protein per tablespoonful)

FASTEST TOMATO SAUCE

Phases 1/2/3 Ⓥ
Preparation: 10 minutes / Cooking: 20 minutes

This is so quick and easy to do and always useful to have on hand, as a quick sauce for 'pasta' and also for making an Open-Faced 'Pizza' Omelette (see p. 195).

MAKES 300ML (10FL OZ)
1 tablespoon olive oil
450g (1lb) tomatoes, quartered
1 garlic clove, peeled and chopped
salt and freshly ground black pepper

1. Heat the olive oil in a saucepan, put in the tomatoes and garlic, cover and cook over a gentle heat for 10–15 minutes, or until the tomatoes have collapsed.

2. Purée the mixture in a food processor. You could then pour it through a sieve if you want a very smooth sauce, but I don't think this is necessary, provided you've liquidised it thoroughly.

3. Season with salt and pepper to taste.

> 12.2g carbs and 4.1g protein for whole quantity
> (0.7g carbs and 0.2g protein per tablespoonful)

COCONUT SAUCE

Phases 1/2/3 Ⓥ

Preparation: 5 minutes / Cooking: 15 minutes

This is another sauce that's really quick and easy to make, and very useful to have in the fridge for almost instant meals. Just heat some hard-boiled eggs, or cubes of tofu, Quorn or seitan in it, for very fast, tasty curries. Snip some fresh coriander leaves over the top, serve with Cauliflower 'Rice' (see p. 262) or just some fresh watercress, and you've got a feast. By the way, do get organic coconut milk if you can – it's so much nicer and has nothing added to the coconut.

MAKES ABOUT 400ML (14FL OZ)
1 tablespoon olive oil
55g (2oz) onion, peeled and finely chopped
2 teaspoons crushed garlic or garlic paste
2 teaspoons grated fresh ginger or ginger paste
½ teaspoon ground turmeric
3 teaspoons curry powder
1 × 300ml (10fl oz) can organic coconut milk
salt and freshly ground black pepper

1. Heat the olive oil in a saucepan, put in the onion, cover and cook gently for 5–7 minutes, until tender.

2. Add the garlic, ginger, turmeric and curry powder, and stir over the heat for a few seconds. Then pour in the coconut milk, and stir again. Cook over a gentle heat for 4–5 minutes, to combine all the flavours – don't let it boil – then season with salt and pepper, and serve.

> 16g carbs and 7g protein for the whole quantity
> (0.6g carbs and 0.3g protein per tablespoonful)

QUICK EGG DISHES

Egg dishes are wonderfully quick and nourishing – and of course eggs are very low in carbs, which makes them ideal for this diet. See also the Cooked Breakfast Dishes section (pp. 151–9) for some omelettes that make equally good quick lunches.

DEVILLED EGGS

Phases 1/2/3
Preparation: 10 minutes / Cooking: 10 minutes

These make a great main course for lunch and are useful to keep in the fridge as a protein-rich snack for hungry moments. They've saved the dieting life of many a vegetarian low-carber.

> **MAKES 12 HALVES**
> 6 eggs
> 6 teaspoons mayonnaise, bought or home-made (see p. 187)
> 1 teaspoon curry powder
> salt

1. Boil the eggs for 10 minutes; cool and remove the shells.

2. Halve the hard-boiled eggs, scoop out the yolks and put them into a bowl. Mash the yolks, then add the mayonnaise, curry powder and salt, and mix to a creamy consistency.

3. Spoon the curry mixture back into the egg whites.

> 0.5g carbs and 6g protein per half egg

EGGS FLORENTINE

Phases 1/2/3
Preparation: 15 minutes / Cooking: 20 minutes

This is a quick egg dish that you can bake in the oven – and you can easily increase the quantities to make it for more people. It would make a very good dinner party starter.

SERVES 1
225g (8oz) baby leaf spinach, rinsed
1 tablespoon olive oil
salt and freshly ground black pepper
2 eggs
55g (2oz) Gruyère cheese, grated

1. Preheat the oven to 180°C (350°F) Gas Mark 4.

2. Cook the spinach in the oil in a saucepan for 1–2 minutes until wilted. Drain and season with salt and pepper.

3. Put the spinach into a shallow casserole dish. Break the eggs on top, season with salt and pepper, then cover with the grated cheese.

4. Bake for about 20 minutes, or until the eggs are done as you like them. Serve at once.

> 4.2g carbs and 36g protein

OPEN-FACED 'PIZZA' OMELETTE

Phases 1/2/3
Preparation: 5 minutes / Cooking: 10 minutes

An open-faced omelette, frittata or tortilla, is another great take on the omelette theme, which in itself offers endless scope for variation. You start it off like a normal omelette, but instead of folding it, leave it open and finish it off under the grill.

SERVES 2
4 eggs
salt and freshly ground black pepper
2 tablespoons olive oil
1 tomato, thinly sliced
1 spring onion, chopped
4–5 black olives
55g (2oz) grated Cheddar cheese

1. Preheat the grill to medium.

2. Beat the eggs with a fork to break them up and combine. Season with salt and pepper.

3. Heat the olive oil in a medium frying pan over a high heat. Pour in the egg mixture and stir it with a fork until it's two-thirds set. Then arrange the tomato slices, spring onion, olives and grated cheese on top.

4. Put the pan under the grill for a few minutes until the omelette has set and the cheese has melted and browned. Serve at once.

6.5g carbs and 41g protein

SPINACH AND GOAT'S CHEESE 'PIZZA' OMELETTE

Phases 1/2/3
Preparation: 5 minutes / Cooking: 10 minutes

Based on a Gordon Ramsay idea, this is very tasty and filling. Try to use 0g carbs goat's cheese if you can – check the label.

SERVES 2
3 tablespoons olive oil
55g (2oz) baby leaf spinach, rinsed
salt and freshly ground black pepper
4 eggs
100g (3½oz) baby goat's cheese with rind, roughly broken into pieces
2 tablespoons freshly grated Parmesan-stye cheese

1. Preheat the grill to medium.

2. Heat 1 tablespoon oil in a pan, add the spinach and cook, uncovered, for a few seconds, until wilted. Remove from the heat, season with salt and pepper, and set aside.

3. Beat the eggs with a fork to break them up and combine. Season with salt and pepper.

4. Heat the remaining olive oil in a medium frying pan over a high heat. Pour in the egg mixture and stir it with a fork until it's two-thirds set. Then arrange the spinach and goat's cheese on top and sprinkle with the Parmesan.

5. Put the pan under the grill for a few minutes until the omelette has set and the cheese has melted and browned. Serve at once.

> 6g carbs and 30g protein

DIPS

A creamy dip, accompanied by some crunchy dippers (see pp. 203–7), is always popular as a starter, snack or part of a salad main meal. There are lots of low-carb possibilities, ranging from something as simple as cream cheese and herbs, for which you don't even need a recipe, to Aubergine and Tahini Dip, which takes a bit of time to make but is well worth the effort. There's even a low-carb version of hummus.

TOFU AND HERB DIP

Phases 1/2/3 **Ⓥ**
Preparation: 5 minutes

This tastes rather like garlic and herb cream cheese. It's quick to make, and great with some vegetable crudités like radishes, strips of red pepper and celery.

SERVES 2
250g (9oz) firm tofu, drained
1 garlic clove, peeled and crushed
several sprigs of parsley
1 tablespoon lemon juice
2 tablespoons chopped chives
salt and freshly ground black pepper

1. Break the tofu into rough chunks and put into a food processor with the garlic, parsley and lemon juice.

2. Whiz until you get a creamy consistency. Then stir in the chives, and season with salt and pepper to taste.

1.4g carbs and 20g protein per serving

SESAME AND TOFU HUMMUS

Phases 1/2/3 Ⓥ
Preparation: 10 minutes / Cooking: 4–5 minutes

This tastes so much like the real thing that people often don't realise it's not! Eat it with low-carb vegetables, such as chicory spears, celery sticks, a few radishes, a few cauliflower florets, one or two button mushrooms. Or make it slightly runnier, by adding a tiny bit more water and lemon juice, and use it as a creamy dressing for a leafy salad.

SERVES 2
40g (1½oz) sesame seeds
½ teaspoon salt
250g (9oz) firm tofu, drained
1 garlic clove, peeled and crushed
2 tablespoons lemon juice
2 tablespoons water
1 tablespoon olive oil (optional)

1. Toast the sesame seeds by putting them into a small pan with the salt and stirring over the heat until they turn light brown and begin to jump around.

2. Remove from the heat and grind to a powder in a coffee grinder.

3. Break the tofu into chunks and put into a food processor with the ground sesame seeds and garlic. Whiz to a thick cream, then add the lemon juice and the water as necessary until you get a lovely creamy consistency.

4. Finally whiz in the olive oil if you wish – it's very nice without it, too – or you could drizzle the olive oil over the top if you prefer.

> 3g carbs and 23g protein per serving

VEGAN CREAM CHEESE

Phases 1/2/3 Ⓥ
Preparation: 5 minutes / Standing time: 1 hour minimum

This is the most delicious cream cheese. You can make it from the soya yogurt described in the Breakfast Dishes section – or you could use shop-bought plain, unsweetened soya yogurt.

MAKES 225G (8OZ)
350g (12oz) plain, live soya yogurt, bought or home-made (see p. 147)
optional flavourings: salt, crushed garlic, freshly ground black pepper, chopped chives

1. Line a sieve with a piece of butter muslin, wide muslin bandage (a roll of 10cm (4in) bandage is useful for this) or kitchen paper. Set the sieve over a bowl.

2. Pour the yogurt into the lined sieve and leave for at least an hour – several hours, or overnight, is best.

3. Remove the cream cheese from the sieve and discard the water in the bowl.

4. Use the cream cheese as it is, or season with salt and other flavourings to taste.

> 8.4g carbs and 15.8g protein for whole quantity

AVOCADO DIP

Phases 1/2/3 Ⓥ
Preparation: 5 minutes

Very simple, but so good. (And such a joy to be able to indulge in this without guilt!)

SERVES 2
1 large ripe avocado
1 tablespoon lemon juice
a few drops of Tabasco
salt and freshly ground black pepper
chopped fresh coriander (optional)

1. Cut the avocado in half, and remove the skin and stone. Cut the flesh into rough chunks and place in a food processor, if you want to make it really smooth, or into a bowl if you want more texture.

2. Add the lemon juice, Tabasco and some salt and pepper, and either whiz or mash to the consistency you want. Mix in some chopped coriander, if using, and serve.

2.3g carbs and 2.5g protein per serving

AUBERGINE AND TAHINI DIP

Phases 2/3 **V**

Preparation: 40 minutes plus cooling time / Cooking: 30 minutes

This creamy, smoky dip, also known as babaganooj, is quite addictive.

SERVES 2–4

2 medium aubergines, pricked all over

2 garlic cloves, peeled and crushed

2 tablespoons pale tahini

2 tablespoons olive oil

2 tablespoons lemon juice

salt and freshly ground black pepper

1. Put a grid shelf from the oven over the top of your cooker so that you can place the aubergines on it, over the burners, to char. Or put them under a hot grill. Either way, it will take about 25–30 minutes and you'll have to turn them frequently – it's quite useful to leave the stalks on, to give you something to hold when you turn them.

2. Let the aubergines cool slightly, then peel off the charred skin: it will come off easily in long strips.

3. Put the aubergines into a food processor with the garlic, tahini, olive oil and lemon juice and whiz to a pale, smooth cream. Season to taste with salt and pepper.

> 40g carbs and 16.4g protein for the whole quantity

BLUE CHEESE DIP

Phases 1/2/3
Preparation: 5 minutes

This is nice with some sticks of celery and radishes for dipping.

SERVES 2
200g (7oz) cream cheese
100g (3½oz) blue cheese, crumbled
a few drops of Tabasco
salt and freshly ground black pepper

1. Put the cream cheese into a food processor with the crumbled blue cheese and Tabasco, and whiz to a cream. Season to taste with salt and pepper.

> 3.9g carbs and 18.3g protein per serving

Vegan variation:
Replace the cream cheese with vegan cream cheese, bought or home-made (see p. 199), and replace the blue cheese with vegan blue cheese.

DIPPERS

As for dippers, most of the traditional vegetable crudités are low-carb enough to be eaten without restrictions but there are crunchy things you can make, too, including those in this section and the crunchy Almond Crackers on p. 296.

Here are some more ideas:

- **Toast**: Cut thin slices of Low-Carb Bread (see p. 294) and toast it. Or toast normal-sized slices, then slit the pieces in half across to make two very thin pieces, which you can put under the grill, uncooked-side up, to make Melba toast.

- **Lovely low-carb vegetables**: Slices of red, green or yellow pepper, spring onions, sticks of celery and cucumber, pieces of cauliflower, raw mangetouts, sticks of turnip, daikon, celeriac or kohlrabi, crunchy radishes – and, in Phases 2 and 3 of the diet, carrot and even some thin slivers of apple.

I DON'T BELIEVE IT'S TOFU

Phases 1/2/3 **V**
Preparation: 10 minutes (plus optional marinating time)
Cooking: 45 minutes

This is the recipe to make for convinced tofu-haters. The tofu is baked with a savoury, crunchy coating and it's very tasty. I usually make at least double this quantity, as it's very popular and equally good hot or cold. Try it hot with mayonnaise, bought or home-made (see p. 187), or Easy Tomato Ketchup (see p. 189), or cold with Tofu and Herb Dip (see p. 197) or Avocado Dip (see p. 200). Nutritional yeast can be found in good health shops and is a very useful ingredient, which keeps well (see Sources and Stockists p. 319 for more details).

SERVES 1–2

1 × 250g (9oz) packet firm tofu, drained and cut into slices about
 5mm (¼in) thick

1 tablespoon carb-free soy sauce

2 tablespoons nutritional yeast

2 teaspoons Italian seasoning herb mix

½ teaspoon dry mustard powder

½ teaspoon garlic powder

½ teaspoon onion powder

olive oil

1. Preheat the oven to 200°C (400°F) Gas Mark 6.

2. Put the tofu on a plate in a single layer, sprinkle the soy sauce over it and leave to marinate while you prepare the coating. (Or leave it for several hours if you have time.)

3. To make the coating, put the nutritional yeast, Italian seasoning, mustard powder, garlic powder and onion powder onto a plate and mix.

4. Dip the slices of tofu into the coating, covering both sides. Place in a single layer on a lightly oiled baking sheet.

5. Bake for about 45 minutes, until golden and crisp, turning them halfway through.

> 4g carbs and 44g protein for the whole quantity

CHEESE CRISPS

Phases 1/2/3
Preparation: 10 minutes / Cooking: 10 minutes

You probably wouldn't want to put the oven on especially for these, but they're a nice treat to make when it's on for something else, and they do keep well in a tin. Trouble is, it's difficult to stop eating them . . .

MAKES 8
40g (1½oz) mild Cheddar cheese, finely grated

1. Preheat the oven to 180°C (350°F) Gas Mark 4.

2. Put 8 little piles of grated cheese well apart on a baking sheet.

3. Place in the oven and bake for about 5 minutes, or until each pile of cheese has spread into a lacy, crisp, golden circle.

4. Allow to cool briefly on the tray, then lift off with a palette knife, blot on kitchen paper, and store in an airtight container.

> 0.2g carbs and just under 1g protein per crisp

CRUNCHY TOFU STICKS

Phases 1/2/3 **Ⓥ**
Preparation: 10 minutes / Cooking: 10 minutes

These are great with a creamy salad, like Coleslaw (see p. 184), or dipped into Sesame and Tofu Hummus (see p. 198), mayonnaise, bought or home-made (see p. 187), or mashed ripe avocado. They also make a good replacement for crisps or tortilla chips, when you feel like something crunchy ... You need to eat them immediately, while they're still crisp, as they don't keep well. For a 'keeping' type of tofu strip, try I Don't Believe It's Tofu (see p. 203).

SERVES 1–2
1 × 250g (9oz) packet firm tofu, drained and blotted dry
olive oil for shallow-frying
salt
1–2 tablespoons finely grated Parmesan cheese or sesame seeds
  (optional)

1. Cut the tofu into long slices about 5mm (¼in) thick – as thin as you can, really.

2. Heat the oil in a frying pan, put in the tofu in a single layer and fry until crisp on both sides, turning when the first side is done. You'll most likely need to do more than one batch.

3. As the slices are done, put them onto a plate lined with kitchen paper and sprinkle with a little salt and the grated cheese or sesame seeds if using.

> 4g carbs and 27g protein for the whole quantity

TOFU FALAFEL

Phases 1/2/3 Ⓥ

Preparation: 10 minutes / Cooking: 10 minutes

I love falafel so I was determined to make a low-carb version – and here it is. I think they're pretty much like the real thing, and packed with protein. They're lovely, hot or cold, with a creamy dip.

SERVES 2

1 × 250g (9oz) packet firm tofu, drained
a small handful, about 15g (½oz), of parsley or coriander
1 garlic clove, peeled and crushed
2 teaspoons ground cumin
1 tablespoon soya protein isolate powder or soya flour
salt
olive oil for shallow-frying

1. Break the tofu into chunks and squeeze each firmly in your hand to extract as much liquid as you can.

2. Put the tofu into a food processor with the parsley or coriander, the garlic and cumin, and whiz to a purée.

3. Sprinkle the soya protein isolate powder or soya flour over the top and whiz again to combine, then season with some salt. Form the mixture into about 10 small balls.

4. Pour enough olive oil into a small frying pan to cover the base by about 5mm (¼in) and heat. Add the tofu balls – if the oil is hot enough they will sizzle immediately when they go in. Fry until brown and crisp all over, moving them around so that all surfaces get into the oil. Don't rush this. It takes about 10 minutes, I find, to get them really crisp. Drain on kitchen paper and serve hot or cold.

> 2.3g carbs and 23g protein per serving

Chapter 11

Main Meals

The recipes in this section are divided into five groups. First there are some tasty 'Grills', then spicy 'Stir-Fries and Curries', followed by 'Pasta' dishes (ingenious low-carb recipes which have all the speed and tastiness of traditional pasta, if not quite the same flavour and consistency). Then there are the warming 'Baked Main Meal Dishes', which make up the largest part of this section and will see you through from quick everyday meals to special occasions; and finally there are some 'Vegetable Side Dishes', including a couple of low-carb 'rice' recipes, a wonderful cauliflower 'mash' and some other specially good vegetable dishes.

GRILLS

I've interpreted the word 'grills' to mean quick, simple, tasty dishes that can be cooked either under the grill, or in a griddle pan on top of the stove – or even on a barbecue. This is the kind of fast, flavoursome food that everyone loves – *and* it's delightfully low in carbs too.

LOW-CARB VEGEBURGERS

Phases 1/2/3 Ⓥ
Preparation: 15 minutes / Cooking: 10–15 minutes

It's easy to make your own delicious, healthy vegeburgers. They freeze well and can be cooked straight from frozen.

SERVES 2
115g (4oz) firm tofu, drained
115g (4oz) frozen vegetarian TVP 'mince' or finely chopped seitan
   (see p. 218)
1 tablespoon soy sauce
salt and freshly ground black pepper
olive oil

1. Whiz the tofu, mince or seitan and soy sauce in a food processor, or with a stick blender, until combined. Taste and season as necessary, and press together into two burgers.

2. Brush the burgers on both sides with olive oil and cook in a griddle pan or under a grill, or on a barbecue, turning to cook the second side. Alternatively, you can fry them in hot olive oil, then drain.

> 3g carbs and 18g protein per burger

CHEESY PORTOBELLO 'STEAKS'

Phases 2/3

Preparation: 15 minutes / Cooking: 15 minutes

These 'steaks' are good served with a green salad.

SERVES 2

4 Portobello mushrooms, washed and blotted dry
1 garlic clove, peeled and crushed
salt and freshly ground black pepper
115g (4oz) Cheddar or Gruyère cheese, grated
olive oil

1. Preheat the grill to medium-high.

2. Put two of the mushrooms, stem side up, on a grill pan. Divide the garlic between the two mushrooms, smearing it over the gills. Season with salt and pepper.

3. Pile the grated cheese on the mushrooms, dividing it equally between them, then top each with one of the remaining mushrooms and press the halves together. Rub the top of the mushrooms with a little olive oil.

4. Grill for about 15 minutes, or until the mushrooms are cooked through. Serve at once.

> 8.8g carbs and 2.0g protein per serving

Vegan variation:

Use vegan cheese – but check the carbs carefully as these do vary according to the manufacturer.

GRIDDLED TOFU FILLETS IN MUSHROOM CREAM SAUCE

Phases 1/2/3

Preparation: 30 minutes / Cooking: 30 minutes

From Phase 2 onwards, you can also make this recipe with Quorn fillets, which are a satisfying meat substitute, but a bit high in carbs for Phase 1. Another variation is to use home-made seitan (see p. 218), instead of the tofu, and fry it in olive oil until crisp, instead of griddling. All these variations are good served with a green vegetable or salad and perhaps some Cauliflower Mash (see p. 260) or Cauliflower 'Rice' (see p. 262).

SERVES 2

For the mushroom sauce:

150g (5½oz) button mushrooms, washed and halved

15g (½oz) butter

3 tablespoons double cream

salt, freshly ground black pepper and grated nutmeg

For the tofu fillets:

2 × 250g (9oz) blocks firm tofu, drained

4 teaspoons garlic paste

olive oil

1. To make the sauce, fry the mushrooms lightly in the butter in a small saucepan, for 5–10 minutes, or until tender. Add the cream and simmer over a gentle heat for 2–3 minutes, or until slightly thickened. Season with salt, pepper and grated nutmeg, and set aside.

2. Cut each block of tofu in half, then slice each half horizontally so that you get four thin slices from each – eight in all. Sandwich these in pairs, using the garlic paste as 'glue', to make four 'fillets'.

3. Brush the tofu fillets all over with olive oil and cook them on a hot griddle, so that they cook through and get marked with black grid lines, turning them to cook on both sides. Alternatively, you can shallow-fry them in olive oil until crisp and golden.

4. When the 'fillets' are done, quickly reheat the sauce and serve with them.

> 5g carbs and 43g protein per serving
> (if using ingredients other than tofu, check the carbs)

Variations:

Vegan variation
Replace the double cream with soya cream.

Other fillings
Other tasty things can be used to sandwich the tofu fillets: pesto, peanut butter or black olive pâté, for instance. Count the carbs.

Quorn variation
If using Quorn fillets, rub them with crushed garlic as well as olive oil before griddling.

Seitan variation
Use seitan just as it is, in chunky pieces, frying it in olive oil until crisp and browned, with or without the addition of some crushed garlic.

TANDOORI TOFU

Phases 1/2/3 **V**
Preparation: 10 minutes (plus 10 minutes–24 hours marinating time)
Cooking: 10–15 minutes

This is quick, spicy and delicious. Serve with some spinach or water-cress and slices of tomato. Spiced Spinach (see p. 268) is a great accompaniment for a special meal.

SERVES 1–2
1 × 250g (9oz) packet firm tofu, drained

For the tandoori spice mixture:
1 garlic clove, peeled and crushed, or 1 teaspoon garlic paste
1 teaspoon crushed ginger, or 1 teaspoon ginger paste
a pinch of hot paprika or chilli powder
½ teaspoon ground turmeric
2 teaspoons ground cumin
1 tablespoon olive oil
1 tablespoon lemon juice
a little salt (to taste)

To serve:
1 tablespoon roughly chopped fresh coriander

1. Cut the tofu into 1cm (½in) cubes. Preheat the grill.

2. To make the spice mixture, put all the ingredients into a bowl and mix together.

3. Toss the cubes of tofu in the spice mixture and stir so that they all get coated. If you have time, you could leave the tofu to marinate in the spice mixture for a few hours but this is not essential.

4. Spread the cubes of tofu out on a grill pan or on a baking sheet that will fit under your grill and cook for 10–15 minutes, until sizzling and crisp, turning them a couple of times.

5. Serve hot and sizzling from the grill, sprinkled with the fresh coriander.

3g carbs and 40g protein for whole quantity

Variation:

Tandoori Halloumi or Paneer
Make in the same way, using either Halloumi or Paneer cheese. Check the package for protein and carb content.

SMOKED TOFU KEBABS WITH PEANUT SAUCE

Phases 1/2/3 **V**

Preparation: 10 minutes / Cooking: 20–30 minutes

I love the combination of the smoky flavour of the tofu and the sweetness of the peanut sauce. Serve with some watercress or a small tomato salad. I rather lazily use jars of ginger and garlic paste for this recipe, though you could of course use the real thing.

SERVES 1

175g (6oz) smoked tofu, drained
salt
a little olive oil (for brushing)
4 metal skewers, or 4 wooden skewers soaked in cold water for
   30 minutes to prevent charring

For the peanut sauce:

2 teaspoons smooth, unsweetened peanut butter
¼ teaspoon ginger paste or grated fresh ginger
¼ teaspoon garlic paste or crushed fresh garlic
1–2 tablespoons water

1. Preheat the grill to high. Cut the block of tofu into four fingers, then cut each of these into four, to make 16 cubes. Thread each block of four cubes onto a skewer, brush with oil and put under the grill, until brown and crisp all over, turning them to do each side of the cubes. This process will take 20–30 minutes. Don't rush it – it's important to get the tofu nice and crisp.

2. Meanwhile, make the peanut sauce by mixing all the ingredients together until smooth and creamy. Set aside.

3. Slip the tofu cubes off the skewers and serve with the sauce.

> 3.3g carbs and 31g protein for whole quantity

STIR-FRIES AND CURRIES

You can make such wonderfully tasty and satisfying dishes with exciting Chinese and Indian flavours – some of the tastiest low-carb dishes of all – and they're not difficult to do. Stir-fries are particularly quick to make but, for extra speed, it's handy to keep some frozen Thai or Chinese stir-fry vegetables in the freezer. Toss these, still frozen, in a little hot sesame or olive oil, add some Thai curry paste and some Marinated Tofu (see p. 219) and you've got an almost-instant meal.

CHINESE VEGETABLE STIR-FRY WITH GINGER AND GARLIC

Phases 2/3 Ⓥ

Preparation: 15 minutes (plus 10 minutes–24 hours marinating time)
Cooking: 10–15 minutes

This is really easy, so don't let the long list of ingredients put you off – the tofu needs a lot of flavouring! Incidentally, you could reduce the carbs by about 3g a serving if you leave out the water chestnuts, though they do give a nice crunchy texture.

SERVES 4

1 × 250g (9oz) packet firm tofu, drained

For the tofu marinade:

2 teaspoons grated fresh ginger or ginger paste

1 garlic clove, peeled and crushed

½ teaspoon Dijon mustard

1 tablespoon roasted sesame oil

2 tablespoons soy sauce

For the stir-fry:
2 tablespoons olive oil
700g (1lb 9oz) bok choy/pak choy, sliced
4 spring onions, sliced
100–150g (3½–5½oz) baby mushrooms, rinsed and dried
1 × 225g (8oz) can bamboo shoots, drained
1 × 225g (8oz) can water chestnuts, drained
salt and freshly ground black pepper

1. Cut the tofu into 1cm (½in) cubes.

2. In a shallow dish, mix together the marinade ingredients. Toss the cubes of tofu in this mixture until they are well coated. Leave to marinate for as long as you can, from 10–30 minutes to 24 hours.

3. Drain the tofu cubes, reserving any marinade liquid, then spread the cubes out on a grill pan and grill until crisp, turning as necessary.

4. When the tofu is nearly done – it takes about 20 minutes – heat the olive oil in a wok or large saucepan and put in all the vegetables.

5. Stir-fry for about 5 minutes, or until the vegetables are just tender. Add the tofu and any reserved liquid and mix gently. Season to taste with salt and pepper, and serve.

8.6g carbs and 14.7g protein per serving

SEITAN (WHEAT PROTEIN)

Phases 1/2/3 Ⓥ
Preparation: 15 minutes / Cooking: 30 minutes

Originally from Japan (where seitan means 'is protein'), seitan is high in protein, low in carbs and very versatile – an excellent food for anyone who's not wheat-intolerant. You can sometimes buy seitan in good health shops but it's quick and easy to make it yourself, using gluten powder. This is the basic recipe and, once made, you can then use the seitan in stir-fries, grills or other recipes, just as you would firm tofu. It's delicious just fried with some garlic (see p. 222), or it can be used in any of the ways you'd use meat, or 'fake' meat. For instance, it can be ground up in a food processor and made into burgers (see p. 209) or used as the basis of a stuffing. It also freezes well.

MAKES ABOUT 325G (11½OZ)
100g (3½oz) gluten powder
1 tablespoon soy sauce
4–5 tablespoons water

For the stock:
425ml (15fl oz) water
1 teaspoon vegetable stock or bouillon powder

1. Put the gluten powder into a bowl. Add the soy sauce and 4–5 tablespoons water and mix; it will become springy and bouncy almost immediately.

2. Knead for 1–2 minutes, then stretch it flat with your hands, fold and roll it. Flatten it again and, with a sharp knife, cut it into small pieces – they will swell as they cook.

3. Make a quick stock by heating the 425ml (15fl oz) water and bouillon powder. When it boils, add the seitan pieces, cover and simmer for 30 minutes. Drain thoroughly – the stock makes good gravy.

4. The seitan is now ready for use.

> 10g carbs and 75g protein for whole quantity
> 3.2g carbs and 23.2g protein for 100g (3½oz)

MARINATED TOFU

Phases 1/2/3 Ⓥ
Preparation: 10 minutes (plus 10 minutes–24 hours marinating time)
Cooking (optional): 20–30 minutes

This tofu is tasty, versatile and very yummy, so it's worth making more than you need, and keeping it for snacks, stir-fries and salads. It's great hot or cold. The longer you keep it, either in the marinade, or after it's been cooked, the more the flavours develop. If you want to have it cold, it's good served with watercress, spring onion, celery sticks and radishes.

SERVES 1–2
1 × 250g (9oz) packet firm tofu, drained
2 teaspoons freshly grated ginger or ginger paste
1 garlic clove, peeled and crushed
½ teaspoon Dijon mustard
2 tablespoons soy sauce

1. Cut the tofu into 5mm (¼in) slices.

2. In a shallow container, mix together the ginger, garlic, mustard and soy sauce. Toss the slices of tofu in this mixture and turn them around so that they are well coated.

3. Leave to marinate for as long as you can, from 10–30 minutes to 24 hours.

4. Eat the tofu slices straight from the marinade, put them on a grill pan and grill until they're sizzling, stir-fry them in a little olive oil until they're crisp, or bake them in a moderate oven for 20–30 minutes.

> 3.3g carbs and 40g protein for the whole quantity

VEGETABLES AND SMOKY TOFU WITH SATAY SAUCE

Phases 2/3 Ⓥ
Preparation: 15 minutes / Cooking: 10–15 minutes

This is a wonderfully filling and tasty dish, packed with protein and special enough, I think, to serve non-veggy friends.

SERVES 2

1 × 220g (8oz) packet smoked tofu, drained
olive oil
225g (8oz) baby mushrooms, washed and halved
1 red pepper, de-seeded and chopped
400g (14oz) bok choy/pak choy, roughly chopped
4 spring onions, washed and sliced
1–2 teaspoons toasted sesame oil (optional)
a dash of soy sauce
salt and freshly ground black pepper
chopped fresh coriander (to serve)

For the satay sauce:

3 tablespoons smooth, unsweetened peanut butter
4 tablespoons water
1 garlic clove, crushed
1 teaspoon grated ginger
1 tablespoon soy sauce
a dash of Tabasco sauce or a pinch of chilli powder

1. Cut the tofu into 1cm (½in) cubes and fry in a little olive oil until golden and crisp all over. Remove from the frying pan and keep warm.

2. Heat a little more oil in the frying pan if necessary and fry the mushrooms and red pepper for about 10 minutes, or until cooked.

3. Meanwhile, simmer the bok choy/pak choy in boiling water for 2–3 minutes, until just tender. Drain, and add the tofu, mushrooms, red pepper and spring onions, toasted sesame oil if using, a dash of soy sauce, salt and pepper to taste, and stir-fry over the heat for 2–3 minutes, to combine everything and give the flavours a chance to blend. Just before serving, scatter the chopped fresh coriander over the vegetables and tofu.

4. Meanwhile, make the satay sauce. Mix all the sauce ingredients together in a bowl until you get a fairly smooth, thick consistency. Reheat gently in a small saucepan or serve cold, with the vegetables and tofu.

14g carbs and 32g protein per serving

GARLIC-FRIED SEITAN

Phases 1/2/3 Ⓥ

Preparation: 15 minutes / Cooking: 10–15 minutes

Once you've made a batch of seitan, try this – it's the quickest and, I think, one of the nicest things to do with it, resulting in chewy, garlicky 'nuggets', which you can eat with a sauce and vegetables, or as a savoury snack. They also freeze well and can be reheated in the oven or under the grill from frozen.

MAKES ABOUT 325G (11½OZ)

1 tablespoon olive oil
15g (½oz) butter
1 quantity Seitan (see p. 218)
2 garlic cloves, peeled and crushed
salt and freshly ground black pepper

To serve:
a few slices of lemon
mayonnaise, bought or home-made (see p. 187)

1. Heat the oil and butter in a large frying pan. Put in the seitan pieces and fry over a moderate heat until golden-brown all over, stirring as necessary.

2. Add the garlic and stir-fry for 1–2 minutes longer. Season to taste with salt and pepper and serve with lemon slices and mayonnaise.

> 12g carbs and 75g protein for whole quantity
> 3.2g carbs and 23.2g protein for 100g (3½oz)

MARINATED TOFU STIR-FRY

Phases 1/2/3 **V**

Preparation: 10 minutes (plus 10 minutes–24 hours marinating time)
Cooking: 5 minutes

This is a lovely, quick stir-fry. You can use your own Marinated Tofu (see p. 219) or you could use bought marinated tofu. If you buy it, be sure to check the carbs, and also the quantity. With one popular make, whereas you get 250g (9oz) in a packet of plain tofu, you get 225g (8oz) if it's smoked, and only 180g (6oz) if it's marinated. So you get a lot more for your money if you buy plain tofu and marinate it yourself . . .

SERVES 2
1 tablespoon olive oil
500g (1lb 2oz) bok choy/pak choy, washed and sliced
4 spring onions, chopped
200g (7oz) baby mushrooms, washed and halved
250g (9oz) marinated tofu, bought or home-made (see p. 219)
salt and freshly ground black pepper

1. Heat the olive oil in a large saucepan or wok, put in all the vegetables and stir-fry for a few minutes until cooked. Then stir in the tofu and cook for a further few minutes to heat through. Season to taste with salt and pepper, and serve.

> 7.8g carbs and 27g protein per serving

THAI COCONUT CURRY ✓

Phases 2/3 **V**
Preparation: 15 minutes / Cooking: 20 minutes

This is quite an unusual way to make a Thai curry – boiling the vegetables rather than stir-frying them – but I prefer to do this to compensate for the richness of the coconut milk. The result is very good, I promise you.

SERVES 2
1 × 250g (9oz) packet firm tofu, drained
1–2 tablespoons Thai red curry paste
2 tablespoons olive oil
1 red pepper, de-seeded and cut into 1cm (½in) pieces
100g (3½oz) baby sweetcorn
4 spring onions, chopped
200g (7oz) bok choy/pak choy, washed and sliced
200g (7oz) mangetouts
1 × 400g (14oz) can organic coconut milk
1–2 tablespoons lime or lemon juice
salt and freshly ground black pepper
2 tablespoons chopped fresh coriander

1. Cut the tofu into 5mm (¼in) slices and spread each slice with red curry paste on both sides, using about 1 tablespoonful of paste.

2. Heat the olive oil in a frying pan and fry the tofu slices on both sides until golden. Remove from the frying pan and keep warm.

3. Bring about 2cm (1in) water to the boil in a saucepan and put in the red pepper, sweetcorn, spring onions and bok choy/pak choy. Cover and cook for about 4 minutes, or until the vegetables are almost tender. Then put in the mangetouts and cook for a further 30–60 seconds.

4. Drain the vegetables and return to the pan, with the tofu and coconut milk. Bring to the boil, stirring gently.

5. Stir in the lime or lemon juice. Taste, and stir in a little more red curry paste if you wish, depending on how hot you like it, and salt and pepper. Sprinkle with the chopped coriander and serve.

> 38.6g carbs and 62.4g protein for the whole quantity
> 19.3g carbs and 31.2g protein per serving

QUICK EGG CURRY

Phases 1/2/3
Preparation: 10 minutes / Cooking: 20 minutes

This is really good served with Cauliflower 'Rice' (see p. 262), or some steamed bok choy/pak choy. And if you have a batch of coconut sauce and some hard-boiled eggs ready in the fridge, you can make it in moments. It's also very easy to adapt this recipe for one person – using two eggs and 100ml (3½oz) coconut sauce – or for four people, using the full quantity of sauce and eight eggs.

> **SERVES 2**
> 4 hard-boiled eggs, halved
> ½ quantity (200ml (7fl oz)) Coconut Sauce (see p. 192)
> 2–3 tablespoons chopped fresh coriander
> sprinkling of hot paprika (optional)

1. Put the eggs into a saucepan or shallow casserole, cover with the sauce and heat gently, in a saucepan or microwave, until piping hot.

2. Scatter with chopped fresh coriander, and some hot paprika if you wish, and serve immediately.

> 4g carbs and 14.4g protein per serving

Vegan variation:
Surprisingly enough, this is also very good if you replace the eggs with plain, firm tofu, cut into cubes; bought, marinated tofu (check the carbs); or some garlic seitan (see p. 222).

QUICK CURRIED TOFU

Preparation: 10 minutes / Cooking: 15–20 minutes

Here's another quick, easy and delicious curry, which I've adapted from *The Protein Powered Vegetarian* by Bo Sebastian. Try it with some Cauliflower 'Rice' (see p. 262) or just a little watercress or green salad.

SERVES 2
1 × 250g (9oz) packet tofu, drained and thinly sliced
4 tablespoons mayonnaise, bought or home-made (see p. 187)
1 teaspoon curry powder

1. Preheat the oven to 180°C (350°F) Gas Mark 4.

2. Put the tofu slices into a shallow casserole dish.

3. Mix the mayonnaise and curry powder together and spoon over the tofu, moving the slices around so that they all get coated.

4. Bake for 15–20 minutes and serve.

2g carbs and 20g protein per serving

Vegan variation:
Replace the mayonnaise with low-carb vegan mayonnaise, bought or home-made (see p. 187).

CHILLI BEANS

Phases 2/3 Ⓥ

Preparation: 15 minutes (plus 1 hour soaking time)
Cooking: 1½ hours

I know this isn't a curry – but it's certainly warming and spicy and so I've included it in this section. Black soya beans can be made into an excellent chilli. You can soak them in cold water overnight, or do the 'quick soak' described here. Try this with some green salad, chopped red pepper, soured cream and avocado.

SERVES 4

200g (7oz) black soya beans
1 onion, peeled and chopped
2 red peppers, de-seeded and chopped
1 tablespoon olive oil
1 garlic clove, peeled and crushed
2 × 400g (14oz) cans tomatoes
chilli powder
salt and freshly ground black pepper

1. Put the beans into a saucepan, cover generously with cold water and bring to the boil. Boil for 2 minutes, then remove from the heat and leave to stand and soak for 1 hour.

2. Drain the beans, cover with fresh water and simmer for about an hour, or until tender.

3. Fry the onion and red peppers in the olive oil in a large saucepan for 10 minutes.

4. Add the garlic, tomatoes, drained beans and chilli powder to taste. Simmer for 15 minutes, to cook the tomatoes, then season with salt and pepper, and serve.

17g carbs and 17g protein per serving

PASTA DISHES

Many vegetables can stand in for pasta, including courgettes, cabbage, and Chinese leaves, all of which can be cut into ribbons. There are also bean sprouts, which make a nice noodle-replacement in Asian-type dishes. Bean sprouts have the advantage of being particularly low in carbs (under 0.7g per 100g (3½oz), or under 2g for a good bowlful). All the other vegetable pasta replacements in this section come to about 8g carbs for a 225g (8oz) serving, which is still relatively low.

There is a kind of grater that you can buy in the US, called a Spiral Slicer, which will cut vegetables such as kohlrabi and turnips into long, spaghetti-like strands. This will add further variety to your 'pasta' dishes if you can get hold of one.

Then there is spaghetti squash, which looks like a normal butternut squash. You simply halve or prick it and cook it in boiling water, or roast it in the oven, until tender. Then you break open the skin and ease out the spaghetti-like flesh with a fork.

You can also buy noodles made from pure soya at Asian shops. They are called shiratake noodles and I'm told they are excellent, though so far I've failed to find them! Keep your eyes open in health shops and supermarkets because, with the increasing interest in low-carb eating, soya pasta is bound to become available soon (but watch out for worthless products stuffed with preservatives and other additives you don't want).

Many of the pasta sauces in this section are quite low in protein (the luscious Vegan Alfredo Sauce is a notable exception) so, unless you're using soya pasta, which will provide plenty of protein, you can make it up by adding grated cheese or by following your pasta with a protein-rich pudding or shake.

COURGETTE RIBBON PASTA WITH MUSHROOMS AND CREAM

Phases 2/3

Preparation: 10 minutes / Cooking: 10 minutes

I love wide pasta ribbons – pappardelle – with a creamy mushroom sauce, and this is a very satisfying low-carb version. It's not high in protein – if you want more of that, you could simply add mushrooms to Cyndi's Vegan Alfredo Sauce (see p. 232).

SERVES 2

450g (1lb) medium courgettes, about 225g (8oz) each, washed and trimmed
olive oil

For the sauce:

1 tablespoon olive oil
15g (½oz) butter
225g (8oz) button mushrooms, washed and halved
1 garlic clove, peeled and crushed
4 tablespoons double cream
salt, freshly ground black pepper and grated nutmeg

1. Start with the sauce. Heat the olive oil and butter in a pan, put in the mushrooms and cook for 3–4 minutes, then stir in the garlic. Add the cream and bubble over the heat for 2–3 minutes until slightly reduced. Season to taste with salt, pepper and grated nutmeg. Set aside.

2. Bring half a saucepan of water to the boil. Meanwhile, cut the courgettes into long, thin ribbons by running a potato peeler down the length of each courgette. Put the strips into the boiling water, bring back to the boil and cook for 2 minutes, or until *al dente*. Drain immediately and return to the pan.

3. Reheat the sauce. Either add the sauce to the courgettes and mix well, or toss the courgettes in a little olive oil, serve out onto plates and top with the mushroom mixture.

8g carbs and 7g protein per serving

Vegan variation:

Replace the double cream with soya cream.

'FETTUCINE' WITH CYNDI'S VEGAN ALFREDO SAUCE

Phases 2/3 Ⓥ
Preparation: 15 minutes / Cooking: 10–15 minutes

Cyndi's Vegan Alfredo Sauce, which I've adapted just slightly by using almonds instead of cashews, is wonderful: really creamy and delicious, and packed with protein. It's great with vegetable 'pasta' and I also like it with Roasted Vegetables (see p. 265) and Roasted Cauliflower with Lemon (see p. 267). You can use it whenever you want to add some extra protein to a meal. If you can get daikon (a long, white radish), it makes lovely 'fettucine' and is very low in carbs – but you can also use courgettes, turnips or kohlrabi, for varying, slightly higher carb counts (see the Carb and Protein Counter on p. 312).

SERVES 2
500g (1lb 2oz) daikon
olive oil

For the sauce:
1 × 250g (9oz) packet firm tofu, drained and broken into rough pieces
1 garlic clove, peeled and crushed
55g (2oz) flaked almonds
4 good sprigs basil
2 tablespoons lemon juice
100–150ml (3½–5fl oz) water
salt and freshly ground black pepper

1. Start with the sauce. Put the tofu and garlic into a food processor and whiz until smooth. Then add the almonds and basil and whiz again until as smooth as possible.

2. Add the lemon juice and enough of the water – or more – to get a creamy consistency. Season to taste with salt and pepper, transfer to a saucepan and set aside.

3. Bring half a saucepan of water to the boil. Meanwhile, cut the daikon into long, thin ribbons by running a swivel potato peeler down the length.

4. Put the ribbons into the boiling water, bring back to the boil and cook for about 4 minutes, or until *al dente*. Drain immediately and return to the pan.

5. While the daikon is cooking, gently reheat the sauce.

6. To serve, either add the sauce to the daikon and mix well, or toss the daikon in a little olive oil, serve out onto plates and pour the creamy sauce over the top.

7g carbs and 29g protein per serving

CABBAGE TAGLIATELLE WITH RED PEPPER AND ARTICHOKE HEARTS

Phases 2/3
Preparation: 15 minutes / Cooking: 10–15 minutes

A pale green, pointed cabbage is a good type to use – for instance 'Sweetheart' in the summer, or 'January King' in the winter. One cabbage is likely to weigh 500–600g (1lb 2oz–1lb 5oz), once the outer leaves have been trimmed off, and is enough to serve two people.

SERVES 2
1 green cabbage
1 red pepper, de-seeded and halved
1 × 250g (9oz) can artichoke hearts, drained and sliced
a few basil leaves
15g (½oz) pine nuts
salt and freshly ground black pepper
olive oil

To serve:
55g (2oz) grated Parmesan-style or Cheddar cheese

1. Trim the cabbage and cut into long shreds.

2. Put the pepper onto a grill pan, rounded side up, and put under a hot grill for about 10 minutes, or until the skin has loosened and blackened in places. Set aside to cool.

3. Bring half a pan of water to the boil, put in the cabbage and bring back to the boil. Then cook, covered, for 2–4 minutes, until *al dente*. Drain immediately and return to the pan.

4. While the cabbage is cooking, cut the pepper into long strips – there's no need to remove the skin unless you want to.

5. Add the pepper strips, artichoke hearts, basil leaves and pine nuts to the cabbage; season well with salt and pepper. Add a little olive oil if you wish, and serve immediately.

17g carbs and 17g protein per serving

Vegan variation:

Replace the grated Parmesan-style or Cheddar cheese with vegan Parmesan cheese.

SPAGHETTI SQUASH WITH GARLIC CREAM CHEESE

Phases 2/3

Preparation: 15 minutes / Cooking: 35 minutes

Spaghetti squash is fun to use and makes a nice change, but if you can't get this, or want a lower-carb dish (8.8g carbs per serving) you can use 450g (1lb) cabbage instead, as in the recipe on p. 234.

SERVES 2

1 × 900g (2lb) spaghetti squash
1 × 150g (5½oz) packet Boursin cream cheese with garlic and herbs
salt and freshly ground black pepper

To serve:

chopped parsley
55g (2oz) finely grated Parmesan-style cheese

1. Bring a large pan of water to the boil. Prick the spaghetti squash in several places, then put into the boiling water, cover and cook gently for 30 minutes, or until the squash is tender when pierced with a skewer. (Alternatively, halve it and bake in a moderate oven for 20 minutes, or until tender; or use a microwave.)

2. When the squash is tender, use a cloth to hold it, halve it if you haven't already, and scoop out the 'spaghetti' into a saucepan. The carb count given is based on a total of 400g (14oz) scooped-out squash.

3. Add the Boursin to the squash and stir gently to melt the cheese and coat all the strands. Season, scatter with some chopped parsley and serve immediately, accompanied by the grated cheese.

> 11g carbs and 2g protein per serving

Vegan variation:

Replace the Boursin with vegan cream cheese, bought or home-made (see p. 199), mixed with herbs and a little crushed garlic, and serve with grated vegan 'Parmesan' cheese.

BEAN SPROUT 'PASTA' WITH FRESH TOMATO AND BASIL SAUCE

Phases 2/3
Preparation: 15 minutes / Cooking: 25 minutes

Bean sprouts make a surprisingly good pasta substitute. I like them particularly as a noodle replacement in Asian-style dishes, but they also work with western ingredients, as in this recipe. (You could also try them with pesto or with garlic cream cheese, as in other recipes in this section.) I think this recipe is nicest made with fresh tomatoes, though it's OK to use canned ones if you prefer.

SERVES 2
olive oil
1 small onion, peeled and finely chopped
1 garlic clove, peeled and crushed
225g (8oz) fresh tomatoes, peeled and chopped, or ½ × 400g (14oz) can tomatoes
600g (1lb 5oz) bean sprouts
salt and freshly ground black pepper

To serve:
a few sprigs of fresh basil, torn
55g (2oz) grated Parmesan-style cheese

1. To make the sauce, heat 1 tablespoon olive oil in a saucepan, put in the onion, cover and cook gently for 7–10 minutes, until tender. Stir in the garlic and tomatoes and continue to cook, uncovered, for a further 5–10 minutes.

2. For the 'pasta', bring half a pan of water to the boil, drop in the bean sprouts and bring back to the boil. Then cook, covered, for 4–5 minutes, until *al dente*. Drain immediately and return to the pan.

3. Season the sauce with salt and pepper and either add it to the bean sprouts in the pan and serve; or toss the bean sprouts with a little olive oil and seasoning, serve out onto two plates and pour the tomato sauce over the top.

4. Either way, scatter with the torn basil leaves and serve with the grated Parmesan cheese.

9g carbs and 10g protein per serving

RUNNER BEAN SPAGHETTI WITH PESTO

Phases 1/2/3

Preparation: 15 minutes / Cooking: 5 minutes

You wouldn't believe what a good spaghetti-replacement runner beans are, if they're cut straight down into long pieces, getting maybe four to each bean. I bought some already cut like this, just to experiment, and found them to be one of the best pasta-replacements of all.

SERVES 2

400g (14oz) 'traditionally cut' runner beans or 500g (1lb 2oz)
    unprepared runner beans
2 tablespoons pesto
salt and freshly ground black pepper

To serve:

55g (2oz) grated Parmesan-style cheese

1. If the runner beans have not been prepared, cut off the 'strings' from each side, using a sharp knife, then cut each runner bean lengthways from top to bottom, to make long, thin slices, like spaghetti, getting maybe four from each bean.

2. Bring half a pan of water to the boil, put in the bean strips and bring back to the boil and simmer, uncovered, for about 4 minutes, or until *al dente*.

3. Drain immediately, return to the pan and stir in the pesto. Serve onto hot plates and hand round the grated Parmesan cheese.

> 6.5g carbs and 10g protein per serving

Vegan variation:

Use vegan pesto and vegan Parmesan-style cheese, in place of their non-vegan equivalents.

BAKED MAIN MEAL DISHES

These are wonderfully warming and satisfying dishes and include some which I consider to be everyday low-carb basics, such as the Low-Carb Pizza (great to have in the freezer), the Spinach and Cream Cheese Gratin (so quick), the amazingly authentic Mushroom Quiche (which I'm very proud of!), the Roasted Red Peppers with Feta, the Nut Roast with Lemon Sauce (an excellent freezer standby when frozen in slices), as well as great stew (Tofu Cacciatore), a low-carb lasagne – and others.

PARMIGIANA

Phases 2/3
Preparation: 20 minutes / Cooking: 20–30 minutes

This is rich and delicious, and it's fine to use the cheap block kind of Mozzarella. Serve it with some watercress or cooked green beans. Incidentally, you can reduce the carbs in this recipe by 6g a serving (to 9g carbs) if you use 300g (10½oz) courgettes instead of the aubergine. This may not be the traditional Italian dish, but it's still very good, and a nice saving of carbs.

SERVES 2
1 medium aubergine
2 tablespoons olive oil
250g (9oz) canned tomatoes
1 garlic clove, peeled and crushed
salt and freshly ground black pepper
200g (7oz) Mozzarella cheese, finely sliced
a few fresh basil leaves
55g (2oz) grated Cheddar or Parmesan cheese

1. Preheat the oven to 200°C (400°F) Gas Mark 6.

2. Cut the aubergine lengthways into thin slices – try to get nine if you can. Brush the cut sides with olive oil, spread out on a grill pan, and grill until golden-brown and tender, turning them to brown the second side.

3. Meanwhile, purée the tomatoes in a blender or food processor, and mix with the garlic and some salt and pepper.

4. Brush a shallow gratin dish with any remaining olive oil and put three pieces of aubergine in the base, to cover it. Spread with just over a third of the tomato mixture, top with fresh basil leaves, then half the Mozzarella.

5. Repeat the layers, then cover with the remaining aubergine and tomato mixture, and top with the grated cheese.

6. Bake for 20–30 minutes, until golden-brown and bubbling.

15g carbs and 30g protein per serving

Vegan variation:

Replace the Mozzarella cheese with plain tofu, thinly sliced, and use vegan Cheddar-style cheese. This works well, although the texture isn't as 'melting'.

ROASTED RED PEPPERS WITH FETA

Phases 2/3
Preparation: 15 minutes / Cooking: 45 minutes

These are lovely served with some Cauliflower Mash (see p. 260) and a green salad. Incidentally, you can reduce the carbs a bit (by about 2.5g a serving) if you use Brie cheese instead of Feta, for a nice variation.

SERVES 2
2 red peppers, preferably the pointed Ramero kind
olive oil
115g (4oz) Feta cheese, diced
4 cherry tomatoes
4 teaspoons pesto

1. Preheat the oven to 200°C (400°F) Gas Mark 6.

2. Halve the peppers, cutting through the stems as well if you can. Scoop out any seeds and place the peppers side by side in a lightly oiled shallow casserole dish.

3. Distribute the Feta cheese and cherry tomatoes between the four pepper halves, then drizzle a teaspoon of pesto over the top of each.

4. Bake, uncovered, for about 45 minutes, until the peppers are tender and the cheese golden-brown. Serve at once.

11g carbs and 12g protein per serving

Vegan variation:
Use vegan Feta-style cheese and vegan pesto.

SPINACH AND CREAM CHEESE GRATIN

Phases 1/2/3
Preparation: 15 minutes / Cooking: 25 minutes

Keep some frozen chopped spinach in the freezer and you can make this recipe in an instant. I find the best way to drain all the excess water off the defrosted spinach is to squash it into a fine-mesh sieve with the back of a spoon.

SERVES 2
280g (10oz) frozen chopped spinach, defrosted
85g (3oz) Boursin garlic and herb cream cheese
115g (4oz) Cheddar cheese, grated

1. Preheat the oven to 180°C (350°F) Gas Mark 4.

2. Mix the spinach with the cream cheese and half the grated cheese. Spoon the mixture into a shallow casserole and sprinkle the rest of the grated cheese on top.

3. Bake for about 25 minutes, or until golden-brown.

> 4g carbs and 11g protein per serving

Vegan variation:
Use bought or home-made vegan cream cheese (see p. 199) and vegan Cheddar-style cheese – but check the carbs carefully, as these do vary according to the manufacturer.

STUFFED PEPPERS WITH SOURED CREAM AND WALNUT SAUCE

Phases 2/3

Preparation: 30 minutes / Cooking: 55 minutes

Serve these tasty peppers with Cauliflower Mash (see p. 260) or Cauliflower 'Rice' (see p. 262) and a cooked green vegetable or salad.

SERVES 2

1 small onion, about 55g (2oz), peeled and chopped
olive oil
2 green peppers
115g (4oz) frozen vegetarian mince or finely chopped seitan (see p. 218)
1 garlic clove, peeled and crushed
1½ teaspoons ground cinnamon
salt and freshly ground black pepper
150ml (5fl oz) vegetable stock

For the sauce:

150ml (5fl oz) soured cream
15g (½oz) walnuts, chopped

1. Preheat the oven to 180°C (350°F) Gas Mark 4.

2. Fry the onion in 1 tablespoon olive oil, covered, for about 7 minutes, or until tender.

3. Slice the tops off the peppers and set aside – these will be used later as 'lids'. Scoop out the core of each pepper and rinse away the seeds. Stand the peppers in a greased casserole dish – one with a lid if possible.

4. Add the vegetarian mince or chopped seitan to the onion, along with the garlic, cinnamon and salt and pepper to taste.

5. Divide the mixture between the peppers, filling them generously and replace the pepper 'lids'.

6. Pour the stock into the casserole and cover with a lid or foil. Bake for 45 minutes, or until the peppers are tender.

7. Serve with a sauce made by mixing the soured cream or yogurt with the chopped walnuts and seasoning to taste with salt and pepper.

15g carbs and 14g protein per serving

Vegan variation:

Replace the soured cream with soya yogurt, bought or home-made (see p. 147).

SAVOY CABBAGE LASAGNE

Phases 2/3

Preparation: 20 minutes / Cooking: 55 minutes

For this dish, tender Savoy cabbage leaves are layered, lasagne-style, with a tasty tomato, celery, almond and red wine filling, plus Mozzarella and Cheddar cheese. It's very satisfying, wonderful when you're catering for a crowd, and, unlike many lasagnes, is quite quick to make.

SERVES 6

1 Savoy cabbage
1 tablespoon olive oil
1 small onion, peeled and finely chopped
2 garlic cloves, peeled and crushed
2 × 400g (14oz) cans tomatoes in juice
1 × 400g (14oz) can celery hearts, drained and roughly chopped
75ml (2½fl oz) white or red wine
2 teaspoons dried oregano
2 teaspoons dried basil
175g (6oz) almonds, finely ground
salt and freshly ground black pepper
200g (7oz) Mozzarella, sliced
150ml (5fl oz) soured cream
140g (5oz) Cheddar cheese, grated

1. Preheat the oven to 200°C (400°F) Gas Mark 6.

2. Half-fill a large saucepan with water and bring to the boil. Remove the leaves from the cabbage and cut each one in half, discarding the hard stem from each leaf. Plunge them into the boiling water, bring back to the boil, then let them cook for 4–5 minutes, until very tender. Drain well.

3. Meanwhile, heat the oil in another saucepan and fry the onion for about 7 minutes, until tender. Add the garlic, tomatoes and

celery hearts, chopping the tomatoes roughly with a spoon. Add the wine, oregano and basil, then leave to simmer, uncovered, for 15–20 minutes, or until some of the liquid has evaporated.

4. Remove from the stove and stir in the ground almonds. Season to taste with salt and pepper.

5. Line a large shallow casserole dish, about 23 × 29cm (9 × 11½in), with a good layer of cabbage leaves. Spoon half the tomato mixture on top, then cover with the Mozzarella slices. Put more cabbage leaves on top, then the remaining tomato mixture. Top with the rest of the cabbage. Pour the soured cream evenly over the cabbage and sprinkle with the grated Cheddar cheese.

6. Bake for about 25 minutes, or until golden-brown. Cut into 6 portions, using a sharp knife. Then lift each one out, using a fish slice.

14g carbs and 25g protein per serving

NUT ROAST WITH LEMON SAUCE

Phases 1/2/3
Preparation: 20 minutes / Cooking: 60 minutes

This makes a big nut roast because I think it's a useful dish to make for a crowd, and also to freeze in individual slices. The quantities can easily be halved, if you wish, to make enough to fill a 450g (1lb) loaf tin. Also, of course, you don't have to serve it with the rich lemon sauce, although it's a wonderful addition for a special occasion. Alternatively, you could have it with a creamy yogurt and fresh herb sauce (chopped chives, tarragon, parsley and anything else you fancy just folded into plain yogurt with some seasoning). It also slices beautifully when cold and then it's good with some mayonnaise, bought or home-made (see p. 187).

NOTE: It's best to use the vegan mayonnaise (see p. 188) instead of the lemon sauce if you are pregnant or feeling at all unwell, due to the barely-cooked egg yolks in the lemon sauce.

MAKES 12 SLICES, SERVING 6–8 GENEROUSLY
1 medium onion, roughly chopped
250g (9oz) celery stalks, roughly chopped
2 tablespoons olive oil
500g (1lb 2oz) almonds, finely ground
3 eggs
2 teaspoons dried tarragon
juice of 1 lemon
salt and freshly ground black pepper

For the lemon sauce:
250g (9 oz) butter, cut into chunks
4 egg yolks
grated rind and juice of 1 lemon

1. Preheat the oven to 180°C (350°F) Gas Mark 4. Line a 900g (2lb) loaf tin with non-stick paper to cover the base, and butter the sides.

2. Put the roughly chopped onion and celery into a food processor and chop very finely, then fry in the oil, covered, for about 10 minutes, until tender. (Chopping them finely in the food processor speeds up this process.)

3. Put the onion and celery mixture back into the food processor with the ground almonds, eggs, tarragon and lemon juice, and whiz to a smooth purée. Season with salt and pepper.

4. Spoon the mixture into the loaf tin and smooth the top. Bake for 45–60 minutes, until firm.

5. When the nut roast is nearly ready, make the sauce. Melt the butter over a gentle heat, without browning. Put the egg yolks, lemon rind and juice, and some salt and pepper, into a food processor or the goblet of a blender and whiz for 1–2 minutes until thick. Then pour the butter on top, in a steady stream, while still processing or blending slowly.

6. Turn the nut roast out, cut into lovely thick slices and serve with the lemon sauce.

> 4.1g carbs and 10.6g protein per slice
> sauce: 0.7g carbs and 10.8g protein for the whole quantity

TOFU CACCIATORE

Phases 2/3 Ⓥ

Preparation: 15 minutes / Cooking: about 1 hour

I have adapted this recipe for 'hunter's tofu' from *The South Beach Diet Cookbook* by Arthur Agatston. It's quick to prepare and very tasty because the tofu absorbs the flavours as it cooks. I serve this with some lightly cooked broccoli, Cauliflower Mash (see p. 260) or a green salad.

SERVES 2

3–4 tablespoons olive oil
1 × 250g (9oz) packet firm tofu, drained and cut into strips about
    5mm (¼in) thick
1 small onion, peeled and finely chopped
½ red pepper, de-seeded and chopped
½ green pepper, de-seeded and chopped
1 garlic clove, peeled and crushed
1 × 400g (14oz) can tomatoes, chopped
½ teaspoon dried basil
½ teaspoon dried oregano
a pinch of allspice
salt and freshly ground black pepper
a few juicy black olives (optional)

1. Preheat the oven to 200°C (400°F) Gas Mark 6.

2. Heat 2–3 tablespoons of olive oil in a saucepan or frying pan and fry the strips of tofu until they're golden-brown on both sides. Put them in a shallow casserole dish in a single layer.

3. Heat another tablespoonful of olive oil in the saucepan and add the onion, peppers and garlic. Fry for about 5 minutes, without browning. Then add the tomatoes, basil, oregano, allspice and salt and pepper to taste. Cook for a further 5 minutes, remove from the heat and pour the tomato mixture over the tofu in the casserole dish.

4. Put into the oven, uncovered, and bake for about 45 minutes, until the peppers are tender.

5. Serve garnished with a few black olives if you wish.

14g carbs and 24g protein per serving

MUSHROOM QUICHE

Phases 1/2/3
Preparation: 45 minutes / Cooking: 1 hour

This is delicious – the almond pastry tastes just like a light whole-meal shortcrust.

SERVES 6
For the almond pastry:
225g (8oz) almonds, finely ground
55g (2oz) butter
½ teaspoon salt

For the filling:
15g (½oz) butter
1 tablespoon olive oil
500g (1lb 2oz) mushrooms, washed and sliced
3 garlic cloves, peeled and crushed
salt and freshly ground black pepper
3 eggs, beaten
4 tablespoons double cream

1. Preheat the oven to 180°C (350°F) Gas Mark 4.

2. To make the pastry, mix the ground almonds, butter and salt together until they form a dough – this can be done in a food processor.

3. You can simply press the dough into a 20cm (8in) flan tin or dish. Or you can roll the dough out between two sheets of non-stick baking paper, peel off the top piece of paper and invert the rolled dough over the tin. You then press it into the tin, through the paper, before peeling off the final layer of paper.

4. Trim the edges of the pastry by pressing them down lightly to fit the dish – there need not be any pastry left over because it's soft enough to press it into position.

5. Prick the base of the flan all over and bake in the oven for 15 minutes, until set and golden brown. Set aside, and turn the oven setting down to 170°C (325°F) Gas Mark 3.

6. Make the filling by heating the butter and olive oil in a saucepan, adding the mushrooms and garlic, and cooking, uncovered, for 10–15 minutes, until the mushrooms are tender and any liquid has boiled away. Season to taste with salt and pepper.

7. Spread the mushroom mixture evenly in the base of the flan. Whisk together the eggs, cream and some salt and pepper, and pour over the mushrooms.

8. Bake for 45 minutes, until set. Serve hot, warm or cold, cut into 6 pieces.

5g carbs and 14g protein per serving

LOW-CARB PIZZA

Phases 1/2/3
Preparation: 30 minutes / Cooking: 30 minutes

This is surprisingly good. Amazingly, it turns out very much like a real pizza, though of the soft-crust rather than the crisp-crust variety. Half-fat cheese is used because it gives the best result. The slices of pizza freeze well and can be heated from frozen.

MAKES 6–8 PIECES

SERVES 2
200g (7oz) half-fat Cheddar cheese, grated
115g (4oz) low-fat cream cheese
3 eggs
½ teaspoon dried oregano
1 garlic clove, peeled and crushed
225g (8oz) tomatoes, washed and quartered
salt
½ can artichoke hearts, sliced
½ green pepper, thinly sliced
2–3 tablespoons finely grated Parmesan cheese
8 black olives

1. Preheat the oven to 190°C (375°F) Gas Mark 5.

2. Line a 13 × 9cm (5 × 3½in) Swiss roll tin with non-stick baking paper. Sprinkle the grated Cheddar cheese evenly into the tin so that the paper is covered.

3. Beat together the cream cheese, eggs, oregano and garlic. Pour this mixture over the cheese, moving the cheese as necessary so that it all gets covered with the creamy mixture.

4. Bake for 30 minutes until firm to the touch and golden-brown.

5. Put the tomatoes into a shallow casserole dish and put them into the oven too, uncovered. Or simmer them in a saucepan for about 15 minutes, until soft and collapsed. Liquidise or beat the tomatoes to make a sauce and season to taste with salt.

6. Spread the tomato sauce over the pizza base, then arrange the artichoke hearts and thin slices of pepper on top, sprinkle with the Parmesan cheese and finish with the black olives. Bake for 10 minutes, and cut into 6 or 8 pieces.

> If cut into 6 pieces, each contains 4.3g carbs and 15g protein
> If cut into 8 pieces, each contains 3.2g carbs and 11g protein

ASPARAGUS 'QUICHE'

Phases 1/2/3
Preparation: 10 minutes / Cooking: 25 minutes

This is a crustless quiche – perfect for all stages of low-carbing, and one of my favourites. (For a quiche with a crust, which is great for the later stages of the diet, see p. 253.)

SERVES 4
250g (9oz) asparagus, trimmed and cut into 5cm (2 in) lengths
salt and freshly ground black pepper
6 eggs, whisked
salt and pepper
175g (6oz) Gruyère cheese, finely grated

1. Preheat the oven to 180°C (350°F) Gas Mark 4.

2. Cook the asparagus in a little boiling water for a few minutes until it's just tender; drain and place evenly in a quiche dish. Sprinkle with half the grated cheese.

3. Whisk the eggs with some salt and pepper. Pour over the asparagus and cheese, then top with the remaining cheese.

4. Bake for 25–30 minutes, or until set, risen and lightly-browned.

5. Serve hot, warm or cold.

> 3g carbs and 25g protein per serving

Vegan variation:

ASPARAGUS 'QUICHE'

Phases 1/2/3

Preparation: 10 minutes / Cooking: 25 minutes

Here is a vegan version of the crustless Asparagus Quiche ...

SERVES 4

250g (9oz) asparagus, trimmed and cut into 5cm (2in) lengths

175g (6oz) vegan Cheddar cheese finely grated – look for one with
 very few carbs, see p. 313

350g (12oz) plain tofu, drained and broken into chunks

½ teaspoon turmeric

3 tablespoons plain unsweetened soya milk

salt and pepper

1. Preheat the oven to 200°C (400°F) Gas Mark 6.

2. Cook the asparagus in a little boiling water for a few minutes until it's just tender; drain and place evenly in a quiche dish. Sprinkle with half the grated cheese.

3. Whiz the tofu in a food processor with the turmeric, soya milk and some salt and pepper, until smooth and creamy. Pour over the asparagus and cheese, allowing the mixture to spread to the edges, then top with the remaining cheese.

4. Bake for 25–30 minutes, or until set, risen and lightly-browned.

5. Serve hot, warm or cold.

> 1.6g carbs and 7.2g protein per slice

VEGETABLE SIDE DISHES

Vegetables play a big part in the Vegetarian Low-Carb Diet at every stage – and the joy is that nearly all vegetables are suitable, certainly from Phase 2 onwards.

Even during Phase 1 (the Carb Cleanse), you can eat plenty of spinach, chard, bok choy/pak choy, spring greens, Chinese leaves, cauliflower, kale, broccoli, Savoy cabbage and Brussels sprouts.

Other low-carb vegetables are French beans, mangetouts, asparagus, artichoke, chicory and okra. Then there are green and red peppers, aubergines and courgettes . . .

Most of these vegetables can be cooked by the 'water steaming' method: that is, bringing about 1–2.5cm (½–1in) water to the boil in a large saucepan and putting the vegetables on top, then covering. The vegetables half-boil and half-steam. When they're tender to your liking, drain them and toss with a little butter, olive oil or roasted sesame oil, and salt and pepper to taste.

Some vegetables are at their best when roasted. I love to cook aubergines, courgettes, onions and red peppers in this way and there are some recipes for them in this section.

Although potatoes, sweetcorn, beetroot and parsnips are a bit high in carbs for the first two phases of the diet, they can be included occasionally once you reach your goal weight. In the meantime, cauliflower and turnips both make excellent potato substitutes, and celeriac, Jerusalem artichokes, daikon, salsify and kohlrabi (if you can get them) are other delicate and delectable low-carb root vegetables.

CAULIFLOWER MASH

Phases 1/2/3 Ⓥ
Preparation: 15 minutes / Cooking: 10 minutes

This cauliflower mash is a revelation: I really love it, and find it fills the 'comfort food' gap left by mashed potatoes. You can also make lovely mash with turnips, celeriac and kohlrabi – they're all worth a try.

> **SERVES 2–4**
> 1 large 600g (1lb 5oz) cauliflower, broken into florets
> 28g (1oz) butter or 2 tablespoons olive oil
> 2–3 tablespoons unsweetened soya milk
> salt and freshly ground black pepper
> grated nutmeg (optional)

1. Bring 5cm (2in) water to the boil in a large saucepan. Put in the cauliflower florets, bring back to the boil, cover and cook for 5–7 minutes, until the cauliflower is tender. Drain well.

2. Put the cauliflower into a food processor with the butter or olive oil, soya milk and some salt and pepper, and grated nutmeg if using. Whiz until you get a smooth, thick consistency.

3. Return to the saucepan and gently reheat, stirring so that it doesn't catch, then serve.

> 20g carbs and 12g protein for the whole quantity

Variation:
For a more luxurious version, replace the soya milk with 2–3 tablespoons double cream (1.2g carbs) or soya cream (1.5g carbs), along with the butter or olive oil.

THREE CHEESE CAULIFLOWER GRATIN

Phases 1/2/3
Preparation: 15 minutes / Cooking: 15 minutes

This could be a side dish with a grilled vegeburger or a main dish, accompanied by a green salad and some Low-Carb Bread (see p. 294).

SERVES 2
300g (10½oz) cauliflower
1 teaspoon Dijon mustard
15g (½oz) butter or ½ tablespoon olive oil
2 tablespoons low-carb mayonnaise, bought or home-made (see p. 187)
2 tablespoons double cream or soya cream
55g (2oz) Brie cheese, diced
55g (2oz) Gruyère cheese, grated
salt and freshly ground black pepper
28g (1oz) almonds, finely ground
28g (1oz) Cheddar cheese, grated

1. Cook the cauliflower in a little boiling water until tender – about 5 minutes. Drain and chop roughly.

2. Preheat the grill. Mix the cauliflower with the mustard, butter or olive oil, mayonnaise, cream, Brie and Gruyère cheese and season.

3. Put the mixture into a shallow casserole dish, and sprinkle the top with the ground almonds and the grated Cheddar cheese.

4. Grill for about 5–10 minutes and serve at once.

> 6.1g carbs and 25.8g protein per serving

Vegan variation:
Use olive oil, vegan mayonnaise, soya cream and vegan cheeses – but check the cheese carbs carefully, as these vary according to the manufacturer.

CAULIFLOWER 'RICE'

Phases 1/2/3 Ⓥ
Preparation: 15 minutes / Cooking: 5 minutes

This rice substitute is great for serving with curries, stir-fries and any dish that you'd normally serve with rice.

SERVES 2
½ medium cauliflower, about 300g (10½oz)
salt

1. Grate the cauliflower finely, or chop it in a food processor, so that it's like rice.

2. Cook the 'rice' in 2.5cm (1in) boiling water for 2–3 minutes until tender. Drain well and season to taste with salt.

> 5g carbs and 3g protein per serving

Variation:
For fried 'rice', heat 1 tablespoon olive oil and a knob of butter in a pan, put in the raw cauliflower, and toss it over the heat for 1–2 minutes until it's done.

TVP 'RICE'

Phases 1/2/3 **Ⓥ**

Preparation: 10 minutes / Cooking: 10–15 minutes

Here is another rice substitute, quite different from the cauliflower one but equally good in its own right and particularly useful for serving with a vegetable dish such as Roasted Ratatouille (see p. 266), or a curry, to create a protein-rich meal.

SERVES 2

85g (3oz) TVP (textured vegetable protein) natural 'mince'
1 tablespoon olive oil
a little chopped parsley
1 garlic clove, peeled and crushed (optional)
salt and freshly ground black pepper

1. Cover the TVP with boiling water and set aside for a few minutes to hydrate, then simmer until tender – about 15 minutes.

2. Drain, return to the pan, and add the olive oil, chopped parsley, garlic if using, and some salt and pepper to taste.

3. Reheat gently, and serve.

> 4.5g carbs and 19g protein per serving

TURNIP CHIPS

Phases 2/3 Ⓥ

Preparation: 15 minutes / Cooking: 30–40 minutes

You can make low-carb chips using turnips, celeriac or kohlrabi (this gives the lowest carbs). They don't taste quite the same, and they don't get crisp, but they look quite similar. And if you fancy chips they can fill that gap and are fun to eat.

SERVES 2
550g (1lb 4oz) turnips, kohlrabi or celeriac, peeled
2 tablespoons olive oil
salt

1. Preheat the oven to 220°C (425°F) Gas Mark 7.

2. Cut the vegetables into strips, put the strips on a baking sheet, add the olive oil and toss to coat. Spread them out in a single layer and bake for 30–40 minutes, turning them halfway through the cooking time.

3. Sprinkle with salt and serve.

> 12.5g carbs and 2.5g protein per serving

Variation:

Turnip Roast Potatoes
You can make these in exactly the same way but cut the turnips into chunky pieces instead of into strips and cook them for a bit longer – about 40–50 minutes.

ROASTED VEGETABLES

Phases 2/3 **V**
Preparation: 10 minutes / Cooking: 45 minutes

These are so easy – just put them into the oven and forget about them until they're done. Serve them with protein in some form: cubes of tofu, which could be baked with the vegetables, perhaps first marinated (as on p. 219), Satay Sauce (see p. 220); Vegan Alfredo Sauce (see p. 232), or some fried Halloumi cheese, or other sliced or grated dairy or vegan cheese. If you want to include an aubergine instead of two of the courgettes, the carbs go up quite a bit (to 18.8 per serving), which is why I've taken to making this all-courgette version.

SERVES 2
3 medium courgettes, cut into 2.5cm (1in) chunks
2 red peppers, de-seeded and cut into 2.5cm (1in) chunks
2 tablespoons olive oil
salt and freshly ground black pepper

1. Preheat the oven to 200°C (400°F) Gas Mark 6.

2. Put the courgettes and peppers into a roasting tin with the olive oil and mix, to coat all the vegetable chunks lightly with the oil. Season well with salt and pepper.

3. Bake, uncovered, for about 45 minutes, until the vegetables are tender and lightly browned. Serve hot, warm or cold.

> 14g carbs and 5.4g protein per serving

ROASTED RATATOUILLE

Phases 2/3 **V**
Preparation: 10 minutes / Cooking: 45 minutes

This is another really easy recipe that you can forget about once it's in the oven. Serve it with grated dairy or vegan cheese, or some TVP 'Rice' (see p. 263), and perhaps a green salad or some cooked cabbage. As with the Roasted Vegetables (see p. 265), I've chosen to make this with extra courgettes instead of aubergine, for a lower-carb total. Using aubergine, instead of two of the courgettes, would boost the carbs in each serving to 22.2g.

SERVES 2

1 medium courgette, cut into 2.5cm (1in) chunks
2 red peppers, de-seeded and cut into 2.5cm (1in) chunks
2 tablespoons olive oil
1 × 225g (8oz) can tomatoes, roughly chopped
salt and freshly ground black pepper
a few sprigs of fresh basil

1. Preheat the oven to 200°C (400°F) Gas Mark 6.

2. Put the courgettes and peppers into a roasting tin with the olive oil, and mix until all the vegetables are lightly coated with the oil.

3. Bake uncovered, for 30 minutes. Then add the tomatoes and return to the oven for a further 15 minutes, or until the vegetables are tender and lightly browned.

4. Tear some basil leaves over the top and serve hot, warm or cold.

> 17.5g carbs and 6.8g protein per serving

ROASTED CAULIFLOWER WITH LEMON

Phases 2/3 Ⓥ

Preparation: 5 minutes (plus optional 12 hours marinating time)
Cooking: 45 minutes

This is a revelation – you'd hardly believe cauliflower could taste this good! Eaten just as it is, sprinkled with salt, it almost makes a French fries replacement, even if it doesn't really look the part. It's also great with some creamy Vegan Alfredo Sauce (see p. 232) – or mayonnaise, bought or home-made (see p. 187), for dipping.

SERVES 2

1 large 600g (1lb 5oz) cauliflower, broken into florets
grated rind of 1 lemon
2 tablespoons lemon juice
2 tablespoons olive oil
salt and freshly ground black pepper

1. Preheat the oven to 200°C (400°F) Gas Mark 6.

2. Put the cauliflower into a roasting tin with the lemon rind and juice and the olive oil, and mix until all the florets are coated. For an extra-special result, you could then leave it overnight to marinate – but this is by no means essential.

3. Bake uncovered, for about 45 minutes, until the cauliflower florets are tender and lightly browned. Sprinkle lightly with salt. Serve hot, warm or cold.

10g carbs and 6g protein per serving

SPICED SPINACH

Phases 2/3 Ⓥ

Preparation: 15 minutes / Cooking: 12–15 minutes

One of my favourite Indian restaurant dishes – here's an easy home version.

SERVES 2

1 small onion, peeled and finely chopped
1 garlic clove, peeled and finely chopped
1 tablespoon olive oil
1 teaspoon cumin seeds
1 teaspoon ground coriander
500g (1lb 2oz) spinach leaves, washed
1 tablespoon lemon juice
salt and freshly ground black pepper

1. Fry the onion and garlic in the olive oil over a gentle heat in a covered pan for 5–7 minutes, until tender. Stir in the cumin seeds and ground coriander, and cook for a further 1–2 minutes.

2. Put in the spinach and cook until it has wilted, stirring from time to time – about 5 minutes.

3. Stir in the lemon juice, season to taste with salt and pepper, and serve.

6.2g carbs and 8g protein per serving

Puddings

Having something sweet at the end of a meal, or even saved for a treat later in the evening, is what enables some people to stay on the Vegetarian Low-Carb Diet for weeks and even months without cheating.

Sara is a very successful low-carber and self-styled 'dessert queen' (you can read her story on p. 59), and she says:

'I need my evening treat and look forward to it during the day. Knowing I'm not depriving myself gives me much-needed will-power to resist other temptations during the day. When I started the diet, during the Carb Cleanse, I used a lot of whipped cream, home-made hot chocolate made with cocoa powder, stevia and soy milk or cream mixed with water, and dessert teas and decaf coffees with dollops of real cream and stevia to sweeten. I would freeze strongly brewed mint tea, sweetened with stevia, for a no-carb sorbet. I ate probably 2000 calories, with over half of them coming from fat. And eating this way lost 80lb in the last year . . . Not bad, even if I do say so myself.'

Although fruits, and of course sugar, have to be restricted when you're low-carbing, you can still have some very delicious and satisfying puddings, as you'll see from the recipes which follow. However, you do need to know your own body – and perhaps even more, your attitude: how you react (mentally as well as physically) to the inclusion of sweet treats.

The more I study the case histories of successful dieters, the more I realise how individual we all are. Foods which seem fine and healthy for some people, and which they can eat while losing weight steadily, seem to bring others to a complete standstill. So my advice about desserts – and even more about baking, in the final section – is to go gently.

Try a dessert or treat that you like the sound of, and which is suitable for your stage of the diet, and see what effect it has. If you find it slows, or stops, your weight loss, you'll be able to make an informed decision next time. Slow but steady weight loss is better than none at all, and if this treat enables you to keep to the diet, then it's most likely worth it. However if it sends you into 'binge mode', it might not be wise to have it too often.

Most people find that their 'sweet tooth' diminishes when they do the Vegetarian Low-Carb Diet; fruits like raspberries and blackberries taste really sweet, and they need less and less sweetener – one of the advantages of this way of eating. However, many of these puddings require some form of sweetener and you will need to consider the pros and cons before deciding which one to use. (For more on this, see pp. 35–8.)

Here are some quick and simple pudding ideas:

- Whipped cream with stevia or low-carb sweetener and vanilla, coffee or cocoa to flavour.

- Home-made Low-Carb Hot Chocolate (see p. 141) with whipped cream on top.

- Black coffee with a dollop of whipped cream on top.

- Strong sugar-free mint, ginger or raspberry tea topped with whipped cream or soya cream.

- Ginger or Mint Sorbet (see p. 272).

- Red Fruit Jelly (see p. 274) with cream.

- Soya or Greek yogurt, with or without a few fruits such as raspberries, strawberries or blackberries.

- Strawberries, blackberries or raspberries with cream.

- Unsweetened canned rhubarb with cream.

- Fruit fool: a low-carb fruit such as raspberries or unsweetened canned rhubarb, folded into whipped double cream and/or thick yogurt, sweetened to taste.

- Home-made low-carb Almond Crackers (see p. 296) and cheese.

- Selection of low-carb cheeses with celery sticks and radishes.

- A bowl of Crunchy Granola (see p. 148).

- Rhubarb Crumble (see p. 284) with cream.

- Chocolate Mousse (see p. 276).

- Creamy Berry 'Yogurt' (see p. 275).

- Pancakes (see p. 158) with raspberries, blackberries and cream.

- A home-made Choc Ice (see p. 278)

COLD PUDDINGS

Some cold puddings, like the sorbets (below), are very light and refreshing and won't add anything to your daily carb total. For instance, many people find Red Fruit Jelly (see p. 274) a great 'diet-saver'. You really can eat as much of this as you like, as it's both carb-free and calorie-free. You can add a dollop of whipped cream or a good swirl of soya cream if you wish, but you will need to count the carbs in these.

Other cold puddings, such as Chocolate Mousse (see p. 276), Creamy Berry 'Yogurt' (see p. 275) or Uncooked Cheesecake with Strawberry Topping (see p. 283) supply useful amounts of protein and can be used to boost the level for a meal, if you've had a relatively low-protein main course, like one of the low-carb pasta dishes (see pp. 230–9).

GINGER SORBET

Phases 1/2/3 ⓥ

Preparation: 15 minutes / Cooking: 10–15 minutes

This is very refreshing and tangy. It's best made in an ice-cream maker if you have one. Alternatively, you can freeze it in a bowl, beating it often to break up the crystals. You can also make it into more of a 'granita' type of dessert by pouring it into small ice-cube moulds, freezing, then pulverising in a food processor – but you do need a good strong processor to do this.

SERVES 2

115g (4oz) fresh ginger root, peeled and cut into chunks
1.2 litres (2 pints) water
stevia or your chosen carb-free sweetener

1. Put the ginger and water into a saucepan and bring to the boil. Then simmer, uncovered, for 20 minutes, until the ginger is

beginning to get tender and the liquid has reduced to about 425ml (15fl oz) and has a strong ginger flavour.

2. Leave to cool, then remove and discard the ginger.

3. Sweeten the ginger liquid to taste with stevia or your chosen sweetener. You'll need about ½ teaspoon pure stevia – more if you're using stevia with bulker. Your taste buds will be the best guide.

4. Freeze in an ice-cream maker according to the maker's instructions, or in the freezer, as described above.

> Trace carbs and 0g protein

Variations:

Raspberry Sorbet
Soak 6 raspberry, strawberry and loganberry tea bags (without any added sugar) in 568ml (1 pint) boiling water. Leave until cold, then squeeze out the tea bags and discard. Sweeten to taste and proceed as above.

Mint Sorbet
Make as described for Raspberry Sorbet, using peppermint tea bags.

RED FRUIT JELLY

Phases 1/2/3 Ⓥ
Preparation: 10 minutes plus cooling and setting time
Cooking: 2–3 minutes

This is a perfect, sparkling jelly and I have to admit, I love it. I use vegetarian gelatine, which can be found in the baking section of large supermarkets. With the product I use, the main ingredient is carrageenan (from a type of seaweed). One sachet is enough to set 568ml (1 pint) liquid, and it has to be mixed with cold liquid, then brought to the boil. You could use other types of vegetarian gelatine – just follow the instructions on the packet.

SERVES 3–4
6 raspberry, strawberry and loganberry tea bags (without any added sugar)
568ml (1 pint) boiling water
stevia or your chosen low-carb sweetener
1 sachet vegetarian gelatine powder or sufficient to set 568ml (1 pint) liquid

To serve:
whipped double cream or soya cream (optional)

1. Put the tea bags into a measuring jug, add 568ml (1 pint) boiling water and leave until cold.

2. Squeeze out the tea bags and discard. Sweeten the liquid to taste with stevia or your chosen sweetener.

3. Put the liquid into a saucepan, sprinkle the vegetarian gelatine on top and whisk until dissolved, then bring to the boil. (Or follow the directions on the packet if different.)

4. Pour into a bowl or individual bowls and leave in the fridge to set. Serve with dairy double cream or soya cream, if using.

Trace carbs and 0g protein per serving
(add extra for cream – 1 tablespoon double cream adds 0.4g
carbs, 1 tablespoon unsweetened soya cream adds 0.2 carbs)

CREAMY BERRY 'YOGURT'

Phases 1/2/3 Ⓥ
Preparation: 2–3 minutes

This is light and creamy, yet filling. You can use frozen berries for an 'ice-cream' version, and can also vary it by adding other ingredients, such as cottage cheese, ground flax seeds (linseeds), chopped almonds and so on – but do count the carbs.

SERVES 1

55g (2oz) frozen summer fruits, defrosted

150ml (5fl oz) unsweetened soya milk, bought or home-made
(see p. 145)

stevia or your chosen low-carb sweetener (optional)

125–140g (4½–5oz) firm tofu

1 tablespoon whipping cream or soya cream

1. Put all the ingredients into a blender, food processor or the goblet that comes with a stick blender, and whiz until thick and creamy.

2. Taste and add the sweetener of your choice if needed: it's quite sweet as it is. Eat at once.

5g carbs and 29g protein

CHOCOLATE MOUSSE

Phases 1/2/3 Ⓥ
Preparation: 10 minutes

Creamy, chocolaty, soothing, easy to make, very low in carbs – and a great source of protein and nourishment to boot. What more do you want from a pudding? You could use silken tofu for this – some people prefer the flavour of this more delicate type – but I find normal tofu works just as well, whizzed with enough soya milk to get a smooth, light texture.

SERVES 2
1 × 250g (9oz) packet plain firm tofu, drained and broken into pieces
2–4 tablespoons unsweetened soya milk, bought or home-made
  (see p. 145)
4 teaspoons cocoa powder
2 tablespoons whipped dairy cream or soya cream
stevia or your chosen low-carb sweetener

To serve:
whipped double cream or soya cream and grated chocolate (optional)

1. Put the tofu into a blender, food processor or the goblet that comes with a stick blender, and whiz very thoroughly, with enough soya milk to get a thick, creamy consistency.

2. Add the cocoa powder and cream, and whiz again, until well blended.

3. Taste and add sweetener of your choice. I find xylitol gives the best results with this – about 2 dessertspoonfuls will sweeten the whole quantity.

4. Spoon into bowls and chill until required. Serve topped with whipped cream, soya cream and/or a little grated chocolate if using.

2.5g carbs and 20g protein per serving
(add extra for cream – a tablespoon of double cream adds
0.4g carbs, unsweetened soya cream 0.2 carbs; a teaspoonful
of finely grated dark chocolate adds about 0.5g carbs)

RASPBERRY ICE-CREAM

Phases 2/3 **V**
Preparation: 3–4 minutes

SERVES 1
85g (3oz) frozen raspberries
150ml (5fl oz) double cream, soya cream or unsweetened soya milk,
   bought or home-made (see p. 145)
stevia or your chosen low-carb sweetener (optional)

1. Put the raspberries, straight from the freezer, into a food processor, blender or the goblet of a stick blender, with the cream, soya
   cream or soya milk.

2. Add some stevia or sweetener to taste, if using, and whiz to a
   thick, creamy ice-cream consistency. Taste, add a little more
   stevia or sweetener if necessary, and eat at once.

8.7g carbs and 3.5g protein

CHOC ICES

Phases 2/3
Preparation: 1¼ hours

This is based on one of Marie Sooklaris' lovely ideas, submitted to the Coconut Discussion Group on the Internet (www.coconut-info.com), and works incredibly well. I love this made with black-berries for the lowest carbs – but strawberries or raspberries are also good. It's important not to miss out the fruit because it helps to prevent the mixture from getting too hard and icy.

MAKES 12
For the ice:
568ml (1 pint) double cream
55g (2oz) ripe blackberries
stevia to taste

For the chocolate coating:
175g (6oz) coconut oil
2 tablespoons cocoa powder
½ teaspoon real vanilla extract
stevia (to taste)

1. Whip the cream until it's thick and holds its shape. Purée the blackberries and stir in – or, if they're very ripe, you could just drop them into the cream when it's about half-whipped, allow-ing them to get mashed by the whisk. Sweeten to taste with stevia. (I use about ⅛ teaspoon of the pure powder – but add it little by little, tasting until you get it right, and remembering that chilling will dull the flavour a bit.)

2. Line a 15 × 25cm (6 × 10in) shallow tin with non-stick baking paper. Spoon the whipped cream into the tin, easing it into the corners and smoothing the top. Mark the top with a knife to form the choc ices – I aim for 12 all together.

3. Put into the freezer until firm – about an hour.

4. Just before it's ready, make the coating. Put the coconut oil into a heatproof bowl over a pan of hot water and stir until it softens – it doesn't need to melt completely.

5. Take the firm ice-cream out of the freezer and pour half of the chocolate coating over the top, tipping the tin so that it runs all over the surface. Put it back into the freezer until set – this only take a few minutes.

6. Then lift the ice and the non-stick paper out of the tin and turn the ice over – you could put it back into the same tin – and peel off the non-stick paper. Pour the rest of the coating over this second side, and put it back into the freezer until the coating is firm.

7. Cut the choc ices through the original lines you made – and eat. You'll be thrilled and amazed.

> 1.7g carbs and 1g protein per choc ice

Vegan Variation:
You can make a very good vegan version by using the Whipped Tofu Topping (see p. 280) instead of cream.

WHIPPED TOFU TOPPING

Phases 1/2/3 **ⓥ**
Preparation: 6 minutes

This is a lovely light topping. You can use it instead of whipped dairy cream, to top puddings and desserts, or you can eat it as a light creamy pudding in its own right. I love it made with flecks of real vanilla. But vanilla extract is also good, or any other flavouring you fancy – coffee, chocolate, lemon. Just include the extra carb or so that these add in your total (see the Carb and Protein Counter, p. 312).

SERVES 2–4
1 × 250g (9oz) packet firm tofu, drained and broken into pieces
5 tablespoons unsweetened soya cream
1 vanilla pod or 1 teaspoon real vanilla extract
stevia (to taste)

1. Put the tofu into a food processor or blender with the soya cream.

2. If you're using a vanilla pod, you can either slit it down the side, scrape out the black gooey seeds and add to the tofu, or you can do what I usually do and chuck in the whole pod (or half the pod if it's a large one). Alternatively, add the vanilla extract if that's what you're using.

3. Whiz until you get a thick, creamy, light, almost 'whipped' consistency. Make sure you process it really thoroughly to achieve this – it must be absolutely smooth, apart from the little flecks of vanilla pod.

4. Add stevia, starting with a tiny speck and increasing until you've got it just right.

5. Serve straight away, or chill.

> 3.1g carbs and 40g protein for the whole quantity
> (0.15g carbs and 2g protein per tablespoonful)

FRUITY ICE LOLLIES

Phases 2/3 Ⓥ

Preparation: 5 minutes, plus cooling and freezing time

It's so good to be able to make a treat that you feel really happy about giving to children – and they can even help make these. Grown-ups may enjoy them, too, on a hot day.

MAKES ABOUT 6, DEPENDING ON LOLLY MOULD SIZE
3 strawberry, raspberry and loganberry fruit tea bags
300ml (10fl oz) boiling water
1 ripe peach, stone removed
100g (3½oz) raspberries
stevia (optional)

1. Cover the tea bags with the boiling water and leave until cold. Then squeeze out all the liquid from the tea bags and discard.

2. Chop the peach roughly, put into a food processor or blender with the raspberries and cold fruit tea and whiz to a smooth purée.

3. Taste and add a little stevia if necessary, then pour the mixture into ice lolly moulds and freeze until solid.

> 2.8g carbs and 0g protein per lolly

SYLLABUB

Phases 2/3
Preparation: 10 minutes

This is a wonderfully luxurious pudding for a special occasion. The finishing touch would be to serve it with some little Crunchy Coconut Biscuits (see p. 308) and a few raspberries.

SERVES 6
568ml (1 pint) double cream, chilled
75ml (2½fl oz) dry or medium white wine
grated rind and juice of 1 lemon
stevia (to taste)
a few toasted flaked almonds

1. Put the double cream into a large bowl with the wine, grated lemon rind and juice, and whisk until thick and fluffy.

2. Stir in a little stevia to taste. Spoon into individual glass dishes and chill in the fridge until required. Decorate each syllabub with a few flaked toasted almonds just before serving.

3.5g carbs and 2.7g protein per serving

UNCOOKED CHEESECAKE WITH STRAWBERRY TOPPING

Phases 2/3
Preparation: 30 minutes (plus chilling time)

This cheesecake, with a creamy topping, is quick and easy to whiz up for a treat. For a classic, low-carb cooked cheesecake, which is difficult to distinguish from the 'real thing', see p. 300.

SERVES 6
100g (3½oz) ground almonds
15g (½oz) butter, softened
400g (14oz) cream cheese
150ml (5fl oz) double cream
grated rind of ½ lemon
1 tablespoon lemon juice
stevia or your chosen low-carb sweetener
225g (8oz) small sweet strawberries, washed, hulled and sliced

1. Mix the almonds and butter together to make a dough (this can be done in a food processor) and press into the base of an 18–20cm (7–8in) loose-based shallow flan tin. This is not a deep cheesecake, so you don't need a tin with a rim any higher than about 1cm (½in). Place in the fridge to chill while you make the topping.

2. Put the cream cheese into a bowl and beat until smooth, then add the double cream and whisk again until very thick and fluffy.

3. Add the lemon rind and juice and stir gently to combine. Sweeten to taste with stevia or sweetener.

4. Spread into the flan tin on top of the almond crust, and chill in the fridge until required.

5. Just before serving, arrange the strawberries on top.

> 5.7g carbs and 9g protein per serving

HOT PUDDINGS

It's amazing what you can make in the way of hot puddings, and how satisfying it can be to eat delicious treats like Rhubarb Crumble and Blueberry Pie while still losing weight! Once you get the hang of using low-carb ingredients, such as finely powdered almonds for flour, and health-giving stevia instead of sugar or sweeteners, there's no end to the delectable treats you can make. Here's just a sample.

RHUBARB CRUMBLE

Phases 1/2/3
Preparation: 15 minutes / Cooking: 10–15 minutes

This is a wonderful recipe for lovers of 'real' puddings. Some supermarkets sell cans of unsweetened rhubarb that can be used in this recipe. This type of unsweetened rhubarb is also excellent on its own, with some whipped cream or soya cream, or it can be mixed with cream to make a fool.

SERVES 4
500g (1lb 2oz) can rhubarb with no added sugar
stevia or your chosen low-carb sweetener
115g (4oz) ground almonds
55g (2oz) butter
a pinch of powdered cinnamon
double cream (optional)

1. Put the rhubarb into a heatproof pudding casserole dish and sweeten to taste with stevia or sweetener.

2. Put the ground almonds, butter and cinnamon into a bowl. Mix with a fork or your fingers to a crumble consistency. Add a little stevia or sweetener to taste, then spoon the crumble on top of the rhubarb.

3. Put under a hot grill for about 5 minutes, or until the crumble is crisp and the rhubarb hot. Serve at once.

4. You could serve a spoonful or two of double cream with this: count the carbs.

5g carbs and 7g protein per serving including the cream

Vegan variation:

Replace the butter with vegan margarine and serve with soya cream instead of double cream.

BLUEBERRY PIE

Phases 2/3
Preparation: 45 minutes / Cooking: 25–30 minutes

This double-crust pie looks and tastes very much like a traditional one. Blueberries are naturally sweet, so they won't need much additional sweetening, but if you want to use a lower-carb filling, try substituting unsweetened canned rhubarb. Red plums also make an excellent filling – remove the stones, simmer the plums in a few tablespoons of water until tender, then sweeten to taste and cool.

SERVES 8

For the pastry:
225g (8oz) ground almonds
55g (2oz) butter, softened
1 teaspoon baking powder

For the filling:
500g (1lb 2oz) blueberries, washed
stevia or your chosen low-carb sweetener

1. Preheat the oven to 180°C (350°F) Gas Mark 4.

2. Mix the ground almonds, butter and baking powder together to make a dough. (This can be done in a food processor if you wish.)

3. Divide the dough in half and pat into a shape that is the same as your pie dish – round, oval, rectangular or square. Put the dough between two sheets of non-stick baking paper and roll out to fit your pie dish. Peel off the top piece of paper and invert the rolled dough over the dish. Press the dough into the dish, through the paper, then peel off the paper.

4. Put the blueberries on top of the pastry and sprinkle them very lightly with stevia (½–1 teaspoon will be plenty) or with your chosen low-carb sweetener.

5. Repeat the rolling process with the remaining piece of dough, ease it on top of the blueberries with the aid of the non-stick paper, press it lightly into position, then peel off the paper. Neaten the pastry with your fingers, pressing in any stray edges. (There's no need to trim off any pastry, as it's so soft you can simply press it into place. Make a steam-hole or two in the crust.)

6. Bake for about 25 minutes, or until the pastry is set, crisp and golden-brown. Serve hot, warm or cold.

6g carbs and 9.3g protein per serving

Vegan variation:

Use coconut oil instead of butter.

LITTLE EGG CUSTARDS

Phases 1/2/3
Preparation: 10 minutes / Cooking: 25 minutes

I use soya cream to make these because it gives a lovely creamy consistency for only a few carbs. These little custards are lovely warm, but I specially like them served chilled, with some whipped cream on top. The coffee variation is particularly good.

SERVES 2
225ml (8fl oz) unsweetened soya cream
2 eggs
½ teaspoon real vanilla extract
stevia or your chosen low-carb sweetener
grated nutmeg (optional)

To serve:
whipped double cream (optional)

1. Preheat the oven to 170°C (325°F) Gas Mark 3.

2. Whisk the soya cream with the eggs, vanilla and a little stevia or sweetener to taste. Pour into two ramekins and sprinkle the tops with grated nutmeg if using.

3. Place the ramekins in a roasting tin and add enough boiling water to come almost to the top of the dishes.

4. Bake for about 25 minutes, or until the custards are set and a skewer inserted into the centre comes out clean.

5. You can eat these hot, warm or cold. If you're serving them cold, top them with some whipped cream for an extra luxurious dessert.

> 2.4g carbs and 10.5g protein per serving
> (add 0.8g carbs if serving with cream)

Variation:

Little Coffee Custards

For this luscious variation, dissolve 1–2 teaspoons espresso coffee granules in the cream and omit the vanilla extract and grated nutmeg.

(add 1 carb per serving for the coffee)

RICOTTA 'RICE' PUDDING

Phases 1/2/3
Preparation: 3–4 minutes / Cooking: 4–5 minutes

As the name suggests, this turns out with a grainy texture and creamy consistency not at all unlike rice pudding – and is nice as a breakfast dish, pudding or comforting snack. It's very quick and easy to make.

SERVES 4
250g (9oz) ricotta cheese
125ml (4fl oz) soya cream
2 eggs

Flavourings:
vanilla extract, grated lemon rind or ground cinnamon
stevia or your chosen low-carb sweetener

1. Put the ricotta cheese, soya cream and eggs into a saucepan. Add flavourings and stevia or sweetener to taste, then whisk or beat well together until creamy.

2. Cook over a gentle heat, stirring all the time, for 4–5 minutes, or until the egg has cooked.

3. Taste and sweeten a little more if necessary, then serve immediately.

3.8g carbs and 11g protein per serving

Baked Treats

Although you can buy an increasing range of low-carb breads, cakes and biscuits, they're expensive and may contain sweeteners and other ingredients that you don't want to eat. But it's easy to make your own – and the results are good, and healthy.

When it comes to low-carb sweeteners, as I've explained before, I like to use stevia for pretty well everything. You have to get it from the US, and it does take a bit of getting used to, but I find the more I use it, the more I love it – a natural, guilt-free sweetener. If that won't do, then my second choice, for occasional use, is xylitol, which is a sugar alcohol obtained from corn. (For more about sweeteners, see pp. 35–8.)

A word of caution here. Low-carb bread, biscuits, cakes and pastries can be really delicious and make wonderful treats that won't upset your diet. But if you over-indulge on them, you'll put on weight just as you would normally. Also, if these are 'trigger foods' for you (see p. 115), the low-carb version may well have the same psychological effect as the non-low-carb version, and send you back to the bingeing/dieting treadmill.

You can buy low-carb flour – but this tends to be expensive and I don't use it. I think finely ground almonds – either bought as 'ground almonds' or the whole brown almonds powdered in a coffee-grinder – make the perfect flour for most baking. (I've also used this to make pastry in other sections of this book.) For recipes where almond flour doesn't seem quite right, I simply use small quantities of soya protein isolate powder.

BREADS

Want to do the low-carb diet but can't do without your bread? Then you *can* have your bread! Here are three nutritious low-carb breads you can make easily at home, a couple of which don't even need yeast. Even the yeast one (my favourite) needs no kneading and can be made in a trice. I like to slice these breads when they're cold, spread them out flat on a cooling rack, freeze them, then store the solid frozen slices in a polythene bag so I can take them out of the fridge individually.

INSTANT MICROWAVE BREAD

Phases 1/2/3
Preparation: 10 minutes / Cooking: 2–3 minutes

This is a quick-to-make, low-carb bread that is high in protein, light in texture and makes great sandwiches and toast.

MAKES 1 SMALL LOAF
150g (5½oz) ground almonds
a pinch of salt
½ teaspoon baking powder
2 tablespoons olive oil
2 eggs, beaten

1. Mix everything together and put into a microwave-safe container.

2. Microwave on full power, uncovered, for 2–3 minutes, or until the bread is risen and firm to the touch and a skewer inserted into the centre comes out clean.

3. Leave to cool on a wire rack.

> 13g carbs and 44g protein for the whole loaf

Variation:

Oven-Baked Version
This same mixture can also be baked in an oven. Double the quantities given and spoon into a 450g (1lb) loaf tin. Bake at 180°C (350°F) Gas Mark 4 for 50 minutes until a skewer inserted into the centre comes out clean. This loaf cuts into 10 slices, each containing about 3g carbs and 9g protein.

WHEAT AND BRAN LOW-CARB BREAD

Phases 1/2/3 (V)

Preparation: 15 minutes (plus 45 minutes for the bread to rise)
Cooking: 45 minutes

This is my version of a recipe I found on the Internet for 'Gabi's World-Famous Bread'. The original recipe involved the use of a bread machine but I couldn't make that work – the automatic kneading produced a very weird loaf. In fact, this bread needs virtually no kneading, as it contains so much gluten. It's very quick and easy to make by hand and results in my favourite low-carb bread – chewy, with a lovely wheaty flavour. A couple of slices of this make a perfect breakfast for toast-lovers *and* supply enough protein to get them through the morning (which is more than you can say for normal toast!).

MAKES 1 X 450G (1LB) LOAF WHICH CUTS INTO 12 SLICES

oil
115g (4oz) wheat gluten powder
85g (3oz) soya protein isolate powder
28g (1oz) flax seeds (linseeds), ground to a powder
55g (2oz) coarse wheat bran
2 × 6g packets 'easy bake' yeast
1 teaspoon salt
3 tablespoons olive oil
250ml (9fl oz) warm water

1. Put the yeast into a small bowl with 2 tablespoons of the water and set aside to dissolve and froth slightly – about 5 minutes. Grease a 450g (1lb) loaf tin generously with oil.

2. Put all the dry ingredients – the wheat gluten, soya protein isolate, ground flax seeds, wheat bran and yeast – into a bowl and add the salt and olive oil.

3. Add water to the bowl and mix gently to get a dough. The gluten soon gets springy, so this bread needs the minimum of mixing and kneading.

4. Form the dough into a loaf shape and put into the greased tin, pushing the dough down in each corner to make a dome-shaped loaf.

5. Cover with a piece of clingfilm and leave in a warm place for 40–45 minutes, until the loaf has risen well above the top of the tin. Meanwhile, preheat the oven to 180°C (350°F) Gas Mark 4.

6. Bake the loaf for 45 minutes. Remove from the tin and leave to cool on a wire rack.

2.2g carbs and 14.6g protein per slice

ALMOND CRACKERS

Phases 2/3 Ⓥ

Preparation: 15 minutes / Cooking: 7–10 minutes

These crackers are wonderful – a savoury snack that anyone would enjoy eating, whether low-carbing or not. It's essential to use non-stick baking paper to roll them out and bake them.

MAKES ABOUT 24 CRACKERS

100g (3½oz) finely ground almonds
½ teaspoon garlic salt
½ teaspoon 'Italian' herb mix
¼ teaspoon chilli powder
freshly ground black pepper
4–6 teaspoons water

1. Preheat the oven to 180°C (350°F) Gas Mark 4.

2. Cut a piece of non-stick paper to line a large baking sheet and then cut another piece exactly the same size. Remove the papers and set aside for the moment. Put the baking sheet in the oven to heat up.

3. Put the ground almonds into a bowl with the garlic salt, herbs, chilli powder and a grinding of pepper, and mix. Then add 4 teaspoons of cold water, and mix to a dough – you could add a tiny bit more water if necessary but be careful not to make it too wet.

4. Form the dough into a rectangle shape and place in the centre of one of the sheets of paper. Put the second piece of paper on top and roll the dough through the paper. Make it as thin as you can, and keep the edges as even as possible, though it doesn't matter if the edges are a bit curved and wobbly.

5. Remove the top piece of paper, and score the dough with a knife to make about 24 crackers. Put the paper of scored crackers onto the preheated baking sheet and bake for 7–9 minutes, until they

are golden-brown and crisp. Look at them after 5–7 minutes. If the crackers at the edges are browning, lift them off with a spatula (they will come off easily) and transfer to a wire rack. Put the rest back in the oven for a few more minutes – but watch them carefully, as they burn easily.

6. You can cool them on the tray or lift them off onto a wire rack. When they are completely cool, store in an airtight container to keep crisp.

8.5g carbs and 21g protein for the whole quantity

CHEESE AND ALMOND BREAD

Phases 1/2/3
Preparation: 15 minutes / Cooking: 50 minutes

This is an easy-to-make, very tasty low-carb bread, which is good as it is, and also toasts well.

> **MAKES 1 X 450G (1LB) LOAF WHICH CUTS INTO 10 SLICES**
> 300g (10½oz) ground almonds
> 1 teaspoon baking powder
> 55g (2oz) butter, softened
> 150g (5½oz) Cheddar cheese, coarsely grated or chopped
> 3 eggs, beaten

1. Preheat the oven to 180°C (350°F) Gas Mark 4. Line a 450g (1lb) loaf tin with non-stick paper, covering the base and sides.

2. Mix the ground almonds and baking powder in a bowl. Add the butter, cheese and eggs, and mix well to combine.

3. Spoon into the loaf tin and bake for 50 minutes until a skewer inserted into the centre comes out clean.

4. Leave to cool on a wire rack, and cut into 10 slices when cold. This bread freezes well – just spread the slices out on a plate or tray and freeze. Then pack them in a container so that you can take them out as you need them.

> 3g carbs and 12g protein per slice

CAKES, BISCUITS AND SWEETS

Yes, you *can* have your cake and eat it on this diet – as long as you count the carbs, that is. And if you're 'spending' your carb allowance on something sweet (or anything else, for that matter), it's got to be worth it, right? Well the treats in this section certainly are, in my opinion, and if you make them as I suggest, with lovely natural stevia to sweeten them, they'll positively do you good as well. Can't say fairer than that ...

BAKED LEMON CHEESECAKE

Phases 1/2/3

Preparation: 15 minutes / Cooking: 45–50 minutes (plus chilling time)

I really love this! It's an excellent cheesecake, very much like a traditional one.

SERVES 8
100g (3½oz) ground almonds
15g (½oz) butter, softened
400g (14oz) cream cheese
2 eggs
150ml (5fl oz) double cream
grated rind of 1 lemon
stevia or your chosen low-carb sweetener

1. Preheat the oven to 220°C (425°F) Gas Mark 7.

2. Mix the almonds and butter together to make a dough (this can be done in a food processor if you wish) and press into the base of a 20cm (8in) spring-release tin.

3. Bake for 10–15 minutes until set and crisp. Remove from the oven and turn the heat down to 180°C (350°F) Gas Mark 4.

4. Beat the cream cheese until creamy, then whisk in the eggs, double cream, lemon and stevia or sweetener to taste. I find 1 teaspoonful of pure stevia powder is right for this, but the types and strengths vary, so it's important to taste, remembering that baking will dull the flavour a little.

5. Pour the filling into the tin, on top of the crisp almond base. Then put the cheesecake in the oven and bake for 35 minutes, until set. Turn off the oven, open the door slightly and leave the cheesecake until cold, if possible.

6. Leave to chill in the fridge until required – overnight is best, if there's time.

> 3g carbs and 8.4g protein per serving

Variation:

If you like a thicker topping – about 2.5cm (1in) – on your cheese-cake, double the quantities of cream cheese, cream, eggs and flavourings, and bake for 1 hour, or until set in the centre. This extra-luscious version will supply 5g carbs and 14g protein per serving.

NUT MUFFINS

Phases 1/2/3
Preparation: 15 minutes / Cooking: 10–15 minutes

This recipe makes eight muffins the size of fairy cakes. Sweeten them to taste – and do try the variation if you like the flavour of chocolate.

> **MAKES 8**
> 40g (1½oz) butter
> 3 tablespoons or 85g (3oz) crunchy peanut butter
> 2 eggs, beaten
> 1 teaspoon baking powder
> 115g (4oz) ground almonds
> 3 tablespoons soya milk, bought or home-made (see p. 145)
> stevia or your chosen low-carb sweetener

1. Preheat the oven to 180°C (350°F) Gas Mark 4.

2. Beat together the butter and peanut butter until creamy, then beat in the eggs.

3. Stir in the baking powder, ground almonds, soya milk and sweetener to taste. (I use ½ teaspoon pure stevia powder.)

4. Spoon the mixture into muffin cases and bake for 15 minutes. Don't over-bake or they will be dry. Leave to cool, and store in an airtight container.

> 2g carbs and 6.3g protein per muffin

Variation:

Chocolate Muffins

For this lovely variation, stir 4 teaspoons unsweetened cocoa into the mixture with the ground almonds and increase the soya milk slightly (by ½–1 tablespoon) to get a soft consistency that holds its shape.

> 2.3g carbs and 6.7g protein per muffin

LOW-CARB BROWNIES

Phases 2/3

Preparation: 15 minutes / Cooking: 10–15 minutes

Although I like to use stevia for most sweetening, there are some recipes where I think xylitol gives a better result, and this is one of them. These brownies have a very delicate, crumbly texture when first made: keep them for 24 hours or so before eating if possible.

MAKES 16 BROWNIES

115g (4oz) butter

100g (3½oz) dark chocolate (with 50% or more cocoa solids)

2 eggs

½ teaspoon vanilla extract

28g (1oz) ground almonds

1 teaspoon baking powder

2 tablespoons xylitol, ½ teaspoon stevia, or low-carb sweetener (to taste)

115g (4oz) chopped walnuts, briefly toasted under the grill before chopping (if you wish)

1. Preheat the oven to 160°C (325°F) Gas Mark 3. Line a 20cm (8in) square tin with non-stick baking paper.

2. Melt together the butter and chocolate in a heatproof bowl, set over a pan of boiling water. Allow to cool slightly, then add the eggs and vanilla and beat until smooth.

3. Stir in the ground almonds, baking powder and xylitol, stevia or sweetener. Taste and check sweetness, adding a little more if required. Stir in the walnuts.

4. Pour into the tin and bake for 15 minutes or until the brownies are risen and set but still slightly gooey in the centre.

5. Cool and cut into 16 pieces.

1.5g carbs and 3g protein per brownie

ALMOND AND LEMON CAKE

Phases 1/2/3
Preparation: 15 minutes / Cooking: 35 minutes

This makes a lovely little cake with a light, moist texture – very much like a normal cake, even though it contains no flour or sugar.

MAKES ABOUT 6 SLICES
85g (3oz) butter, softened
2 tablespoons olive oil
3 eggs
finely grated rind of 1 lemon
200g (7oz) ground almonds
1 teaspoon baking powder
1 teaspoon pure stevia or your chosen low-carb sweetener

1. Preheat the oven to 170°C (325°F) Gas Mark 3. Line a 15–18cm (6–7in) cake tin with non-stick baking paper.

2. Whisk together the butter, olive oil, eggs and grated lemon rind until creamy, then stir in the ground almonds, baking powder and stevia or sweetener.

3. Spoon the mixture into the tin and gently level the top. Bake for 30–35 minutes, until risen and firm to a light touch and a skewer inserted into the centre comes out clean.

4. Leave to cool on a wire rack, then strip off the paper.

> 17.2g carbs and 61.4g protein for the whole cake
> 2.9g carbs and 10.2g protein per slice if cutting into 6 slices

CHOCOLATE ALMOND BARK

Phases 2/3 Ⓥ
Preparation: 15 minutes / Cooking: 10–15 minutes

I love this almond bark, which I've adapted from an original recipe by Marie Sooklaris submitted to the Coconut Discussion Group on the Internet (www.coconut-info.com). It turns out like crisp, nutty chocolate and is an excellent low-carb treat to have when you fancy something chocolaty – both almonds and coconut oil have health-giving properties. (For more about coconut oil, see p. 35.) For this recipe, it's best to grind the almonds yourself. Bought ground almonds are a bit too fine and, without the fibre of the skins, they contain more carbs. If you wish, you can make the chocolate almond bark thicker by using a smaller tin. It will then have a similar consistency to a chocolate bar. However it melts easily so it needs to be kept in the fridge. You can also replace the ground almonds with ground flax seeds (linseeds), which is a good way of getting children to take their vital daily omega oils.

MAKES A 33 X 23CM (13 X 9IN) SHEET
55g (2oz) almonds
85g (3oz) virgin coconut oil
2 teaspoons cocoa powder
stevia or your chosen low-carb sweetener

1. Line a 33 × 23cm (13 × 9in) Swiss roll tin with a piece of non-stick paper. Then place the tin in the freezer to chill while you prepare the mixture.

2. Put the almonds in a coffee-grinder and grind them fairly finely but not to a powder. Spread them out on a baking tin or grill pan and toast under a hot grill for 1–2 minutes until golden-brown.

3. Meanwhile, melt the coconut oil in a saucepan over a gentle heat, taking care not to let it get too hot.

4. Remove from the heat and stir in the cocoa powder, toasted almonds and stevia or sweetener to taste.

5. Pour the mixture into the chilled and lined tin, tipping the tin so that the mixture spreads out thinly, though it won't cover the base completely. Make sure the nuts are fairly evenly distributed.

6. Put into the freezer for a few minutes until it has set. It will then break with a crisp 'snap'. Keep in the freezer, either in the tin or, broken into pieces, in a suitable container.

Variation:

Mint Choc Crisps
Try making this with a few drops of peppermint oil or peppermint flavouring added.

> 5.6g carbs and 13g protein for the whole quantity

CRUNCHY COCONUT BISCUITS

Phases 2/3
Preparation: 15 minutes / Cooking: 20 minutes

These biscuits, which I've adapted from a recipe by Leslie Kenton, are nice to serve with a creamy pudding, for a special occasion, or to offer guests with a cup of tea or coffee. They're a bit like coconut macaroons, with a crunchy outside and slightly gooey centre – rather more-ish.

MAKES 14 BISCUITS
2 egg whites
a pinch of salt
55g (2oz) ground almonds
55g (2oz) unsweetened desiccated coconut
1 teaspoon vanilla extract
1 teaspoon almond extract
1 tablespoon Amaretto or other almond liqueur
stevia powder or your chosen low-carb sweetener (to taste)

1. Preheat the oven to 150°C (300°F) Gas Mark 2. Line a large baking sheet with non-stick baking paper.

2. Whisk the egg whites with a pinch of salt until stiff.

3. Mix together the ground almonds and desiccated coconut, then fold into the egg whites, along with the vanilla and almond extracts, the liqueur if using, and the stevia. (I use ⅛ teaspoon pure stevia, but taste to get it right for you.)

4. Spoon little heaps of the mixture – a bit bigger than a heaped tea-spoonful – onto the baking paper.

5. Bake for 20 minutes, until golden-brown and crunchy on the outside, and a little gooey within. Leave to cool on the baking tray.

0.6g carbs and 1.5g protein per biscuit

KELLY'S DARK CHOCOLATE NUT CLUSTERS

Phases 2/3

Preparation: 5 minutes / Cooking: 10 minutes (plus 30 minutes chilling in fridge)

These are a yummy treat that you can make from normal, dark chocolate. Look for a good-quality one high in cocoa solids – I used one with a minimum of 73 per cent and that's what the carb total is based on. They are quite high in carbs, but great for a special treat with a cup of decaf coffee if you know you can limit yourself to just one – or two!

MAKES 12 CHOCOLATES
½ × 150g (5½oz) block very dark chocolate, broken into squares
a knob of butter
28g (1oz) ground almonds
28g (1oz) desiccated coconut
stevia or low-carb sweetener (to taste)
28g (1oz) pecan nuts, broken into chunks

1. Place a heatproof bowl over a pan of boiling water. Put the chocolate and butter in the bowl and stir together, over the heat, until melted. Add the ground almonds, coconut and stevia to taste – start with ⅛ teaspoonful and gradually increase until you've got it right. Then add the pecan nuts and stir until thoroughly combined.

2. Lay a piece of non-stick baking paper or foil over a shallow baking tray, and drop teaspoonfuls of the mixture onto the paper or foil, flattening each one slightly with the back of the spoon, making 12 in all. Leave to chill in the fridge for about 30 minutes.

3. When the chocolates have hardened, peel them off the paper or foil, and store them in a sealed plastic container in the fridge.

> 2.4g carbs and 1.4g protein per chocolate

Last Words

You've got there – congratulations!

Now I urge you to keep up your enthusiasm by experimenting with new low-carb foods, ingredients and recipes. I've given you as many recipes as I could cram into this book – and I think you'll also find an increasing number of recipes 'out there' as low-carb eating becomes more widely understood and practised.

You might also like to join one of the Internet low-carb discussion groups. My favourite – without the support of which this book would probably not have been written – is LCV (Low-Carb Vegetarian, run by Cyndi Norman, who has taught me so much about vegetarian low-carbing). I recommend it wholeheartedly: it's good to share experiences and recipes with other like-minded people. You'll find details of all these websites at the end of this book (see p. 322) and also the ever-useful Carb and Protein Counter (see p. 312).

And finally, I'd like to leave the very last words to Kathy, who has lost 30lb on the Vegetarian Low-Carb Diet:

'I'm in my late fifties and over the years I've tried many, many diets, unsuccessfully. Now at last, with the Vegetarian Low-Carb Diet, I've found one that works, that I can really stick to. My weight loss hasn't been dramatic – I've lost an average of 2–3lb a week – but it's been steady. I haven't done much exercise, but I've found that walking helps.

'At first, I really missed snacking in the evenings. But I realised that this was my downfall. I wasn't really hungry – one of the joys of this diet is that I've never felt hungry – it was just old habits. Once I realised that, I decided that I wasn't going to let evening snacking spoil my weight loss, and I managed to stop. It was hard at first, but now I don't even think about it, thank heavens.

'I've come to realise that losing weight depends on me, what I think, how I feel, and how determined I am. I've still got more weight to lose, but now I know that, with the right diet and the right attitude, I can do it.'

CARB AND PROTEIN COUNTER

The values given in this table are taken from a number of sources and have been rounded to one decimal place. I believe them to be reasonably accurate but please remember that there will be variation from batch to batch and according to the season and condition of the food. However I hope you will find this table a useful guide. All carbs are 'net' or 'usable', which means that they have already had the fibre subtracted from them.

Ingredient	g per amount given		g per 28g (1oz)		g per 100g (3½oz)	
	Carbs	Protein	Carbs	Protein	Carbs	Protein
Almond butter 5g / 1 tsp	0.9	0.8	5.0	4.3	17.5	15.1
Apple, medium 150g	17.0	0.4	3.2	0.1	11.4	0.3
Artichoke, globe whole 60g	3.5	2.0	1.6	1.0	5.8	3.5
Artichoke, canned hearts, drained 240g	5.0	3.4	0.6	0.4	2.1	1.4
Asparagus			0.5	0.6	1.8	2.2
Aubergine 300g	18.6	2.4	1.8	0.2	6.2	0.8
Avocado 250g	4.5	5.0	0.5	0.6	1.8	2.0
Bamboo shoots 225g can, drained 140g	2.5	2.4	0.5	0.5	1.8	1.7
Basil, dried, ground 1 tsp	0.1	0.1			20.5	14.4
Basil, fresh			0.1	0.7	0.4	2.5
Beans, French			1.1	0.5	3.7	1.8
Beans, runner, stringed			0.7	0.3	2.3	1.2
Bean sprouts			0.2	0.5	0.7	1.8
Beans, whole, green 400g can, 220g drained	3.3	3.3	0.4	0.4	1.5	1.5
Beans, kidney, canned			2.6	1.5	9.2	5.3
Beans, kidney, raw			10.0	6.7	35.1	23.6
Black soya beans, cooked			1.7	2.4	6.0	8.4
Blueberries, fresh			3.4	0.2	12.1	0.7
Blackberries, fresh			1.2	0.4	4.3	1.4
Bok choy / Pak choy			0.3	0.4	1.2	1.5
Bouillon powder 1 tsp	0.3	0.4	4.8	5.2	17.0	18.4
Bran, wheat 1 tbsp	0.8	0.5	6.2	4.4	21.7	15.6
Bread, wholemeal			11.1	2.7	39.2	9.7

Ingredient	g per amount given		g per 28g (1oz)		g per 100g (3½oz)	
	Carbs	Protein	Carbs	Protein	Carbs	Protein
Broccoli 1 head 350g	14.0	9.8	1.2	0.8	4.0	2.8
Brussels sprouts			1.2	1.0	4.2	3.4
Butter					0.1	0.9
Cabbage, Savoy 650g	19.5	13.0	0.9	0.6	3.0	2.0
Cabbage, Chinese USA Pak Choi			0.3	0.4	1.2	1.5
Cabbage, Chinese USA Pe-tsai			0.6	0.3	2.0	1.2
Cabbage, Napa USA			0.6	0.3	2.2	1.1
Carrots			1.9	0.3	6.8	0.9
Cauliflower, trimmed 700g	23.1	14.0	0.9	0.6	3.3	2.0
Celeriac			2.3	0.4	8.1	1.5
Celery stick 62g	0.9	0.4	0.4	0.2	1.4	0.7
Celery hearts 400g can	3.2	2.1	0.3	0.2	1.2	0.8
Cheese, see packets for other varieties						
Cheese, blue			0.7	6.1	2.3	21.4
Cheese, Boursin 150g	0.9	3.0	0.6	2.0	2.0	7.0
Cheese, Brie			0.1	5.9	0.5	20.8
Cheese, Camembert			0.1	5.6	0.5	19.8
Cheese, Cheddar			0.4	7.1	1.3	25.0
Cheese, Cheddar, low-fat			0.5	6.9	1.9	24.4
Cheese, Chèvre blanc			neg	6.5	0.1	23.0
Cheese, cottage			0.8	3.5	2.7	12.5
Cheese, cream			0.8	2.1	2.7	7.6
Cheese, cream, low-fat			2.0	3.0	7.0	10.6
Cheese, Edam			0.4	7.1	1.4	25.0
Cheese, Feta			1.2	4.0	4.1	14.2
Cheese, goat's, soft			neg	6.5	0.1	23.0
Cheese, goat's, semi-soft			0.7	6.1	2.5	21.6
Cheese, Gruyère			0.1	8.5	0.4	30.0
Cheese, Halloumi			0.4	5.7	1.3	20.0
Cheese, Mozzarella			0.6	6.3	2.2	22.2
Cheese, Parmesan			0.9	10.1	3.2	36.0
Cheese, ricotta			1.4	3.2	5.1	11.4
Vegan (Scheese)			0.3	4.1	1.2	14.5

Ingredient	g per amount given		g per 28g (1oz)		g per 100g (3½oz)	
	Carbs	Protein	Carbs	Protein	Carbs	Protein
Chick peas, canned			5.2	1.4	18.2	5.0
Chicory			0.3	0.3	0.9	0.9
Chilli powder 2.6g /1 tsp	0.5	0.3	5.8	3.5	20.5	12.3
Chives, fresh 3g / 1 tbsp	0.1	0.1			1.9	3.3
*Chocolat Patissier, Dark (eg Menier)			8.8	2.3	31.0	8.0
Chocolate, dark, cooking			3.7	3.7	13.2	12.9
Cocoa, 4g (Cadbury's)	0.8	0.8	6.0	5.6	21.0	19.6
Cocoa 1.8g / 1 tsp	0.4	0.35	6.0	5.6	21.0	19.6
Cocoa 5.4g / 1 tbsp	1.1	1.1	6.0	5.6	21.0	19.6
Coconut, desiccated, unsweetened			2.1	2.0	7.4	6.9
Coconut milk 400ml can	11.2	8.0	0.8	0.6	2.8	2.0
Coconut milk, raw			0.9	0.7	3.3	2.3
Coconut oil			0	0	0	0
Coriander seeds 1 tsp	0.2	0.2	3.7	3.5	13.1	12.4
Courgette 200g	4.6	2.4	0.6	0.3	2.3	1.2
Couscous			20.5	4.3	72.3	15.1
Cranberries			2.2	0.1	7.6	0.4
Cream, double 1 tbsp	0.4	0.3	0.7	0.5	2.6	1.7
Cream, whipping 1 tbsp	0.4	0.3	0.8	0.6	2.8	2.1
Cream, fresh, soured			1.1	0.7	3.9	2.6
Cream, soya 1 tbsp	0.2	0.5	0.4	0.9	1.3	3.0
Cream, soya 1 tsp	0.1	0.5	0.4	0.9	1.3	3.0
Cucumber 300g	9.4	2.0	0.9	0.2	3.1	0.7
Cumin seeds 2.1g / 1 tsp	0.7	0.4	9.6	5.0	33.7	17.8
Curry paste, Thai, red 16g / 1 tbsp	0.8	0.4	1.4	0.6	5.0	2.2
Curry powder 6.3g /1 tbsp	1.6	0.8	1.9	3.6	25.0	12.7
Daikon radish	1.0		0.4	0.3	1.2	1.1
Edamame, shelled 90g	6.2	11.1	1.9	3.5	6.9	12.4
Edamame, unshelled 190g total	2.9	5.3	0.9	1.7	3.2	5.9
Eggs, 1 whole 50g	0.4	6.3	0.2	3.6	0.8	12.6
Egg yolk 17g	0.2	2.7	0.3	4.5	0.9	15.9
Egg white 33g	0.2	3.6	0.2	3.1	0.7	10.9

* The carbs in chocolate vary quite a lot – best to check with the manufacturer to be sure.

Ingredient	g per amount given		g per 28g (1oz)		g per 100g (3½oz)	
	Carbs	Protein	Carbs	Protein	Carbs	Protein
Endive			0.2	0.4	0.6	1.3
Fennel bulb			1.2	0.4	4.2	1.2
Flax / linseed 12g / 1 tbsp	0.8	2.3	1.8	5.5	6.4	19.5
Garlic, 1 clove 3g	1.0	0.2	8.8	1.8	31.0	6.4
Ginger, raw 1 tsp	0.3	neg	4.5	0.5	15.8	1.8
Ginger ale			2.5	0	8.8	0
Gluten powder			2.8	21.3	10.0	75.0
Gooseberries			1.7	0.3	5.9	0.9
Green beans			1.0	0.5	3.7	1.8
Kale packet 200g	2.8	6.8	0.4	1.0	1.4	3.4
Kohlrabi			0.7	0.5	2.6	1.7
Lemon juice 1 tbsp	1.2	neg	1.3	0.6	8.2	0.4
Leeks			3.5	0.4	12.4	1.5
Lentils, green			11.3	6.9	39.9	24.3
Lentils, red split			13.2	6.7	46.4	23.8
Lettuce, sweet Romaine			0.3	0.4	1.2	1.2
Lettuce, Iceberg			0.5	0.3	1.8	0.9
Lettuce, red			0.4	0.4	1.4	1.3
Loganberries			2.2	0.4	7.9	1.5
Mayonnaise, Hellmann's 1 tbsp	0.2	0.2	0.4	0.3	1.3	1.1
Melon, Cantaloupe			2.1	0.3	7.3	0.8
Melon, Honeydew			2.4	0.2	8.3	0.5
Melon, Watermelon			2.0	0.2	7.2	0.6
Mustard, plain, made, 1 tsp	0.2		1.0	neg	3.5	neg
Mushrooms, button			0.6	0.9	2.0	3.1
Mushrooms, large flat 110g	2.2	3.4	0.6	0.9	2.0	3.1
Mushrooms, Portobello			1.0	0.7	3.6	2.5
Nectarine 140g	12.3	1.5	2.5	0.3	8.9	1.1
Nuts, almond with skins			2.3	6.0	8.0	21.2
Nuts, Brazil			1.4	4.0	4.8	14.3
Nuts, cashew			7.6	5.2	27.0	18.2
Nuts, hazel			2.0	4.3	7.0	15.0
Nuts, macadamia			1.4	2.2	4.8	7.9
Nuts, peanuts, salted			1.7	7.9	5.9	28.0
Nuts, pecans			1.2	2.6	4.3	9.2
Nuts, pine nuts			2.7	3.9	9.4	13.7

Ingredient	g per amount given		g per 28g (1oz)		g per 100g (3½oz)	
	Carbs	Protein	Carbs	Protein	Carbs	Protein
Nuts, walnuts			2.0	4.3	7.0	15.2
Oat bran			14.4	4.9	50.8	17.3
Oat flour			16.8	4.2	60.0	14.7
Oats			15.8	4.8	55.7	17.0
Okra			1.1	0.6	3.8	2.0
Olive oil			0	0	0	0
Olives, green Queen			0.9	0.3	3.1	1.0
Olives, black, med 1 of 4g	0.2	0.1	1.1	0.3	3.8	1.0
Onion, small 50g	4.4	0.5	2.5	0.3	8.7	0.9
Onion, medium 100g	8.7	0.9	2.5	0.3	8.7	0.9
Onion, large 150g	13.0	1.4	2.5	0.3	8.7	0.9
Onions, spring 1 of 12g	0.6	0.2	1.3	0.5	4.7	1.8
Orange 150g	14.0	1.5	2.7	0.3	9.4	0.9
Oregano, dried 2g / 1 tsp	0.4	0.2	6.1	3.1	21.6	11.0
Papaya / pawpaw, medium 300g	24.0	1.8	2.3	0.2	8.0	0.6
Parsley			0.9	0.8	3.0	3.0
Peach 140g	11.4	1.3	2.3	0.3	8.0	0.9
Peanut butter 16g / 1tbsp	2.1	4.5	3.7	7.9	13.0	28.0
Pear, medium 175g	21	0.6	3.5	0.1	12.4	0.4
Peas, frozen			2.7	1.5	9.5	5.2
Peas, mangetouts 115g	6.0	3.2	1.4	0.8	5.0	2.8
Peppers, green 180g	5.0	1.6	0.8	0.2	2.9	0.9
Peppers, red 180g	7.2	1.8	1.1	0.3	4.0	1.0
Peppers, yellow 180g	9.7	1.8	1.5	0.3	5.4	1.0
Pesto 1 tbsp	1.0	3.0	1.1	3.4	4.0	12.0
Plum, medium 66g	6.6	0.5	2.9	0.2	10.0	0.7
Potatoes, white			3.8	0.5	13.3	1.7
Pumpkin			1.7	0.3	6.0	1.0
Pumpkin seeds			4.0	7.0	13.9	24.5
Quorn			1.6	4.0	5.8	14.0
Radishes			0.5	0.2	1.8	0.7
Raspberries			1.6	0.3	5.5	1.2
Rhubarb, canned 525g	3.7	4.2	0.2	0.2	0.7	0.8
Rhubarb			0.3	neg	1.0	neg
Rice, Basmati			21.5	2.7	76.0	9.6
Rice, brown			20.6	2.1	72.8	7.5

Ingredient	g per amount given		g per 28g (1oz)		g per 100g (3½oz)	
	Carbs	Protein	Carbs	Protein	Carbs	Protein
Rice protein			0.4	3.4	1.6	12.0
Rocket			0.6	0.7	2.1	2.6
Sausages, 2 veggy, grilled	1.8	15.5	0.6	4.9	2.0	17.2
Seitan			0.9	6.6	3.2	23.2
Sesame oil			0	0	0	0
Sesame seeds			3.3	5.0	11.7	17.7
Soya beans, mature raw			5.9	10.3	20.9	36.5
Soya beans, black			3.1	9.1	11.0	23.0
Soya beans, green			1.9	3.7	6.9	13.0
Soya beans, yellow			4.5	10.2	15.8	36.0
Soya cream 1 tbsp	0.2	0.5	0.4	0.9	1.3	3.0
Soya milk, unsweetened Provamel 1 tbsp	0.1	0.6	0.1	1.1	0.4	3.7
Soya protein isolate 28g scoop	0.1	25.0	0.1	25.0	0.4	87.0
Soya yogurt, Sojasun, 250g carton	2.7*		0.7	1.3	2.4	4.5
Spinach, frozen			0.4	1.1	1.2	3.9
Spinach, edible leaves			0.4	0.8	1.4	2.9
Squash, butternut			2.8	0.3	9.7	1.0
Squash, spaghetti, cooked			1.4	neg	5.1	neg
Stevia					neg	neg
Strawberries			1.6	2.0	5.7	0.7
Summer fruits, frozen			1.5	0.2	5.4	0.6
Sunflower seeds			2.3	6.5	8.1	22.8
Swede			1.6	0.3	5.6	1.2
Swiss chard			0.6	0.5	2.1	1.8
Sweetcorn, yellow, raw			4.7	0.9	16.5	3.2
Sweetcorn, mini			2.3	0.5	8.2	1.9
Sweetcorn, baby			0.4	0.7	1.3	2.5
Tahini 15g / 1 tbsp	1.2	4.4	2.3	8.2	8.0	29.0
Tangerine, medium 115g	12.0	0.9	3.3	0.2	11.5	0.8
Tempeh, soya			6.7	7.7	23.7	27.1
Tofu, Cauldron 250g	2.5	40	0.3	4.5	1.0	16.0
Tomatoes, large 100g			0.8	0.3	2.7	0.9
Tomatoes cherry 11g	0.3	0.1	0.8	0.3	2.7	0.9
Tomatoes, sun-dried			12.3	4.0	43.5	14.1

Ingredient	g per amount given		g per 28g (1oz)		g per 100g (3½oz)	
	Carbs	Protein	Carbs	Protein	Carbs	Protein
Tomatoes, sun-dried in oil			5.0	1.4	17.5	5.1
Tomatoes, whole plum, canned 400g	12.0	4.8	0.9	0.3	3.0	1.2
Tomato purée			3.6	1.3	12.6	4.7
Treacle, black 25g / 1 tbsp	16.0	0.4	18.0	0.5	64	1.7
Turnips			18.0	0.3	4.6	0.9
TVP, dry			3.4	14.2	12.0	50.0
TVP, frozen			1.1	4.4	4.0	15.5
Vanilla extract 1 tsp	0.6	0.0	3.6	0.0	12.7	0.1
Vegeburger quarterpounder	1.8	27.0				
Vegetarian mince, frozen			1.1	4.4	4.0	15.5
Vinegar			0	0	0	0
Water chestnuts 225g can, 140g drained	13.7		2.8	neg	9.8	neg
Watercress			0.2	neg	0.7	neg
Wheat bran 3.5g / 1 tbsp	0.8	0.6	6.2	4.4	21.7	15.6
Wheatgerm 7g / 1 tbsp	1.6	2.0	6.5	7.9	22.9	28
Whey powder 20g scoop	1.0	16.0	1.4	22.7	5.0	80
Wine 75ml glass	5.0	3.3			6.7	4.4
Yeast, nutritional 4g / 1 tbsp	0.6	1.8	4.3	13.0	15	46.0
Yogurt, Greek			1.3*	1.0	4.6*	3.7
Yogurt, plain skim milk			2.2*	1.6	7.7*	5.7
Yogurt, plain whole milk			1.3*	1.0	4.7*	3.5
Yogurt, soya, Sojasun, 250g carton	6*	11.3	0.7*	1.3	2.4*	4.5

* These values show the amounts given in tables, but yogurt that has been fermented with live bacteria will often be lower in carbs than this because some of them will have been transformed from lactose to lactic acid by the lactobacillus.

SOURCES AND STOCKISTS

Ingredients and products

Black soya beans

Buy these dried from Asian shops. Unless you speak Chinese you probably won't be able to understand the instructions on the packet, but they're easy to use. You simply soak them overnight in cold water, then simmer for about 1 hour until they're tender (see p. 32). Look out for canned black soya beans too; they're available in the US but I haven't been able to find them in the UK yet.

Edamame (green soya beans)

These are available, frozen, from Asian shops. Again, the packet is generally indecipherable, to me, at any rate, but cooking is easy: just simmer in boiling water for 3–4 minutes, drain and eat by sucking the beans out of the pods, or shell the beans for use in recipes.

Gluten powder

I'm hoping this will soon become available by the packet in health shops. You can however order it over the Internet, as I do, from www.flourbin.com/index2.htm. The product is excellent and the company is helpful. However you do have to give a minimum order of £10 and pay for carriage on top of that. The gluten powder keeps well – store it in the freezer, if necessary, or find some friends to share the order. For more information, the e-mail address is info@flourbin.com, tel: 01246 850124.

Nutritional Yeast Flakes

This is a protein-rich nutritious seasoning, with a cheesy, nutty taste (though vegan), made from primary inactive yeast without artificial additives or preservatives. The name on the tub is Engevita, it is made by Marigold and is available from good health shops. A little goes a long way and it keeps well.

Soya protein isolate powder

Holland & Barrett do a large 900g (2lb) tub of this, which I find great for baking and cooking. Holland & Barrett have assured me that it's GMO-free although they do not state this on the label because all their products are in fact GMO-free. (They also do a chocolate one but that contains artificial sweeteners.)

My favourite soya protein isolate is Jarrow Formulas Iso-Rich Soy. It's very light and fine-textured, unsweetened, with a delicate natural vanilla flavouring, guaranteed organic (which means there are no chemical residues from the processing) and great for making shakes. However it's only available in a 450g (1lb) tub and is quite pricy because it has to be imported from the US. You can find out more about this, and order it by post if you wish, from Jan Freeman at Vitamin UK, PO Box 98, Manchester M20 6PZ, Freephone 0800 056 8148 (within the UK) or tel: 00 44 161 434 2876 (outside the UK). Jan is very helpful and can also advise you about vitamins and xylitol. Website: www.vitaminuk.com.

Stevia

As mentioned earlier, you can't buy this in the UK because it's illegal for anyone to sell it to you (see www.stevia.net/thesteviastory for more about this). It is however easy to buy from many websites and the ones I've dealt with have been friendly, helpful and efficient.

For stevia with 'bulkers', which adds about 1g carbs per serving, but which some people find is the easiest way to use stevia, and for liquid stevia, which some people like, try the Stevita Company, 7650 US Hwy. 287 #100, Arlington, Texas 76001, USA, tel +(1) 817 483 0044, fax +(1) 817 478 8891.
Website: www.stevitastevia.com.

For pure stevia powder (and dried leaves etc if you want them), try www.emperorsherbologist.com/buy-stevioside.html. I have had some excellent pure stevia from them. I prefer the pure type without bulkers but I suggest you start with really small amounts of different types and see which you like best. I've also heard good things about www.nowfoods.com/?action=itemdetail&item_id=3143.

And you can probably get stevia from www.stevia.net.

Vitamins

Look for a complete, good-quality multivitamin made by a reliable company such as Bio-Care, from good health shops, or from Vitamin UK (see above). I also like LifePak, made by Pharmanex, and obtainable from Chryssa Porter, tel: 020 8542 2949 or e-mail: chryssa@pharmanXcare.com. Chryssa has done the Vegetarian Low-Carb Diet successfully herself and is very helpful and supportive.

Whey powder

I recommend you get a good quality micro-filtered type. I like Solgar Whey To Go in vanilla. (It's also available in chocolate, but this is higher in carbs.) It's not as easy to track down as I'd like, but is available from top-quality health shops. If you like it, the large size works out a lot cheaper. For stockists, contact Solgar Vitamin & Herb Ltd, Aldbury, Tring HP23 5PT, tel: 01442 890355, fax: 01442 890366. Website: www.solgar.com.

Xylitol

Not widely available in the UK at the time of writing but probably obtainable over the Internet. I buy it through Jan Freeman of Vitamins UK, see above.

Books

For more about low-carb diets:
Dr Atkins New Diet Revolution, Robert C Atkins, Vermilion
Protein Power, Dr Michael R Eades & Dr Mary Dan Eades, HarperCollins

For more about carb counts:
The Complete Book of Food Counts, Corinne T. Netzer, CTN

For more about the GI diet and many delicious low-GI recipes:
Fast, Fresh and Fabulous, Rose Elliot, BBC Worldwide
(This is a recipe book rather than a diet book, but contains useful information too.)

Useful Websites

www.fitday.com
For food counts, and calculating your daily carbs.

www.nalusda.gov/fnic/foodscomp/search/
A very useful US site which allows you to find nutritional
information, including carb and protein counts for many foods.

www.coconut-info.com
For information on coconut oil.

www.holisticmed.com/splenda/
For facts about artificial sweeteners.

www.foodrevolution.org/what_about_soy_html, and
www.veganoutreach.org/health/soysafe.html
For facts about the safety of soya.

www.stevia.net/safety.html, and
www.stevia/net/thesteviastory
For facts about stevia.

www.immuneweb.org/lists/lcweb.html
For a very friendly, helpful vegetarian low-carb forum you can join to
exchange information and experiences, and ask questions.

www.roselliott.com
Come and visit me at my site!

Index

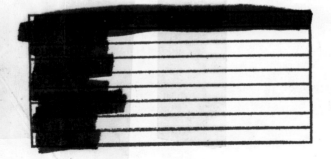